MEDICO-LEGAL ESSENTIALS

Health Records in Court

MEDICO-LEGAL ESSENTIALS

Health Records in Court

JANE LYNCH
LLB
Solicitor

Foreword by

PETER CARTER
General Secretary
Royal College of Nursing

Radcliffe Publishing
Oxford • New York

Radcliffe Publishing Ltd
18 Marcham Road
Abingdon
Oxon OX14 1AA
United Kingdom

www.radcliffe-oxford.com
Electronic catalogue and worldwide online ordering facility.

© 2009 Jane Lynch

Jane Lynch has asserted her right under the Copyright, Designs and Patents Act 1998 to be identified as the author of this work.

British Library Cataloguing in Publication Data

A catalogue record for this book is available from the British Library.

ISBN-13: 978 184619 222 7

The paper used for the text pages of this book is FSC certified. FSC (The Forest Stewardship Council) is an international network to promote responsible management of the world's forests.

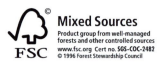

Mixed Sources
Product group from well-managed forests and other controlled sources
www.fsc.org Cert no. SGS-COC-2482
© 1996 Forest Stewardship Council

FSC

Typeset by Pindar NZ, Auckland, New Zealand
Printed and bound by TJI Digital, Padstow, Cornwall, UK

Contents

Foreword

For nurses and other healthcare professionals, an understanding of the law and the way in which it impacts upon their roles, responsibilities and the care they give is becoming an increasingly important part of their everyday work. That's why, in my view, this book is both timely and welcome.

Well written, clear and concise, this book provides useful and practical advice by highlighting real-life case studies and workplace examples. Therefore, it provides a much-needed guide for navigating the complexities and intricacies of medico-legal processes, practices and obligations.

Engaging with the wider factors and issues that shape and influence patient care is essential for all those involved in the delivery of healthcare. I believe this book will not simply provide a practical workplace tool; it will also help to enhance good practice.

Dr Peter Carter
General Secretary
Royal College of Nursing
February 2009

Preface

This book is an essential tool for all those employed in the health sector, which includes doctors, dentists, nurses, midwives, paramedics, allied health professionals, management and administrative staff. Pharmaceutical companies and legal professionals will also find this book useful.

My intention is to enhance good practice, and this book is not designed to teach the health professional to become a lawyer, but to look at practical situations and examine the consequences.

The law has fast become a real challenge for health professionals. The legal climate has changed. To the health professional, the law has become an everyday concern.

The law is a complex area and, not surprisingly, health professionals find it difficult to understand and to apply it in practice. Many books on medico-legal topics tend to jump in with the intricacies of particular statutes. This can often leave health professionals floundering because the basic principles of the law and the way it works are left unexplained. In my student days, I could write an essay on, for example, the role of the magistrate, but it was only when I went back to basics, to understand how the law was made, who else made law, what it consisted of, etc., that I could see the whole picture and it made much more sense. When this understanding is reached, the reasoning becomes clearer and the threads are easier to pull together. Understanding the law is fundamental too when health professionals have to weigh up and make decisions about patient care. So rather than just learning the law verbatim, it is important to understand the thinking behind it. This makes it much easier to apply in practice.

This book seeks to explain the basic legal principles and how they apply in a practical way. The health professional will then be more effective when making decisions in their everyday role. This book explains the legal and professional obligations, best practice in record keeping, professional guidelines, and accountability, and looks at how the court views the records. It is written so that it is easy to understand and answers every day dilemmas using real cases, practical examples and checklists.

Whilst health professionals are aware of their legal and professional obligations to maintain a reasonable standard of records, the practical difficulties they face are:

➤ will the records stand up to legal scrutiny?
➤ what are the consequences of getting it wrong?
➤ how much do I write?
➤ what do I write?
➤ what can I leave out?
➤ can I amend it?
➤ who should write it?
➤ should abbreviations be used?
➤ how do I record telephone advice?
➤ is an email part of the records?
➤ can I write subjective comments, assumptions or opinion?

The examples used are drawn from situations faced by health professionals and real cases. The basic principles should be taken and applied to the health professional's own situation. Throughout the book many questions will be posed for the reader to consider. This is to raise awareness of the issues and to get the reader thinking. There are useful examples and checklists, which may be adapted.

This book does not cover moral and ethical issues.

For ease of reference, throughout the text the phrase 'health professional' is used to include all those involved in healthcare. The word 'patient' is used to include the patient or the client. The word 'he' is used throughout, but is not intended to be derogatory or sexist – it simply provides easier reading.

Jane Lynch
February 2009

About the author

Jane Lynch is a practising lawyer specialising in clinical negligence. She is on The Law Society's specialist clinical negligence panel and is recognised in the Legal 500 as one of the leading practitioners in England and Wales. She is a fellow of the Royal Society of Medicine. Jane is also a legal trainer for the health sector and is involved in training over 250 NHS Trusts, the private health sector and the Ministry of Defence. She is a regular speaker at international conferences and also lectures at several universities on the masters' degree courses. She has had several papers and articles published. Jane is well known in the health sector and is very highly regarded in her field. Jane is a founding director of the Practical Legal Training Agency (www.plta.co.uk), which specialises in legal training for non-lawyers.

Acknowledgements

I am very grateful to all those who contributed to this book. I am particularly grateful to Jane Grove, Lead Community Infection Control Nurse Specialist, for reading the drafts and providing much appreciated guidance and advice.

To my mother, and my daughter, Kate, for their enthusiasm, encouragement, support and patience during my writing of this book.

CHAPTER 1

Introduction to health records

In its 2008 annual report, the National Health Service Litigation Authority (NHSLA) estimated that as at 31 March 2008, its total liabilities of outstanding claims for clinical negligence was £11.9 billion.[1] This includes legal costs and the costs of compensation that was paid out. It does not include the cost of staff and management time in dealing with those complaints, or the additional costs of bed space, which means that the true cost is far higher. The vast majority of clinical accidents arise as a result of a breakdown in communication through poor systems and poor documentation.

Record keeping is a fundamental part of healthcare. Health professionals have both a legal and professional obligation to maintain a reasonable standard of health records. If they fail to do so they will be held accountable. It is therefore important for health professionals to understand their legal and professional obligations, how they apply in practice and what the consequences are of getting them wrong.

If a health professional fails to maintain a reasonable standard of record keeping their accountability will impact in four distinct areas: (i) their patient; (ii) their professional body; (iii) their employer; and (iv) society. This is discussed in detail in Chapter 3.

Health professionals are often concerned about whether their records will stand up to legal scrutiny. In order to put this into context, this book firstly explores the law, accountability and then the records in context. It also specifically covers the courts' view of records.

A good standard of record keeping is the sign of a safe practitioner and helps to protect the welfare of patients. Good records promote high standards of clinical care, continuity of care and better communication between members of the healthcare team. They provide an accurate account of treatment, care planning and delivery and the ability to detect problems at an early stage, such as changes in the patient's condition.

Poor record keeping compromises patient care and often reflects a wider underlying problem with the individual's practice. This makes health professionals vulnerable to legal and professional problems and increases workloads. The vast majority of clinical accidents arising from poor recording keeping and the resulting breakdown of communication and system failures cost the NHS approximately 10% of their annual budget in legal claims.

EXAMPLE OF SYSTEM FAILURE

This was an unreported case involving Mrs S, a 28-year-old woman who was admitted for routine surgery for a prolapsed disc. She was the third patient on the theatre list. The first patient had been operated on and the instruments were being sterilised. The same instruments were required for patient number two and, rather than wait for those instruments to come out of the steriliser, the surgeon swapped the list around. Mrs S then became patient number two. Part-way through the procedure they realised they had forgotten to swap the blood bags over and had administered a wrong blood type transfusion. The patient died on the theatre table.

At the inquest the anaesthetist who had failed to check the wristband with the blood bag explained, 'I am new to the Trust; I trained and worked abroad and we did things differently there'.

The surgeon said, 'Next time I swap the list around I will tell people'.

This is very reassuring! This is a classic example of a system failure and a breakdown of communication. The surgeon tells the theatre nurse, the nurse goes on coffee break and tells someone else, etc., etc., and it then becomes Chinese whispers resulting in a breakdown of communication – in this case with tragic consequences.

Litigation is increasing in relation to consent issues. Sadly, this is not necessarily because valid consent has not been obtained, but rather there is no evidence that valid consent has been obtained. This is because the records are either insufficient in detail or there is nothing recorded. Issues in question often concern what advice was given or risks explained. Consent is a complex area in itself and there is often confusion as to when consent issues should be recorded and how they are recorded. This is explored in more detail in Chapter 7.

There are many reasons why litigation in respect of clinical care has risen in recent years. There have been changes in the law. The Human Rights Act 1998,[2] Data Protection Act 1998[3] and Freedom of Information Act 2000[4] have all impacted on the rights and expectations of the patient. Patients are no longer passive and are much more aware of their rights. They have wider access to information, particularly via the internet. 'No win no fee' arrangements in relation to the legal costs of pursuing a claim are widely publicised. The first thing patients see when they enter a healthcare setting is a leaflet entitled 'How to Complain', which encourages patients to come forward.

Health professionals must be familiar with the law and must uphold the patient's rights. They must also be aware of the issues of consent and confidentiality, amongst other things, and that they are accountable for their actions.

REFERENCES

1 National Health Service Litigation Authority. *Report and Accounts: fact sheet 2, financial information.* London: National Health Service Litigation Authority; 2008.
2 The Human Rights Act 1998.
3 Data Protection Act 1998.
4 Freedom of Information Act 2000.

CHAPTER 2

Health records and the law

Before we look at the records in detail it is important for the health professional to understand their legal and professional obligations in relation to the documentation. We hear words like civil litigation, negligence, breach of duty and accountability. This chapter explains these areas briefly and simply. It is also explains the basic court structure, which places the legal issues in context.

THE COURT SYSTEM

Health professionals may be involved in the court system in many ways: at an inquest, civil proceedings, criminal proceedings or employment tribunal. It may involve matters of a complaint by a patient, or child protection issues. It is highly likely that in all these forums the records will be required and relied upon as evidence.

Further information in relation to the health records used as evidence is explored in more detail in Chapter 18.

SOURCES OF LAW

We know the law exists but most people do not often think about it in their everyday lives even though it is continuously in operation; for example, when goods are bought and sold, when people get married or companies are formed. The law lays down rules in respect of all of these matters. When things are done in the usual way there is little reason to worry. In the normal course of events, people begin to consider the law only when some uncertainty or difficulty arises. When a person looks into their situation after a difficulty has arisen they may find it is probably too late. The law, by its nature, applies retrospectively. It is usually after something has gone wrong that the law steps in.

Everyday decisions are made about patient care, planning and treatment. Health professionals go about their daily routines and, whilst terms like accountability and responsibility form part of their everyday vocabulary, they do not sit back and think 'what does it really mean?' But when something goes wrong they become accountable. Being forewarned is being forearmed and understanding the law and accountability will help health professionals make the right decisions.

The health professional must know the area of law that affects them. For example, those working in mental health should be familiar with The Mental Health Act 1983,[1] Mental Capacity Act 2005[2] and other legislation. Remember, ignorance of the law is no defence.

Very broadly speaking, the law is a set of rules. The law in England and Wales is made up of statutes and common law. (Common law is sometimes referred to as case law.)

Statutes

A statute is law set out in an Act of Parliament, declaring, commanding or prohibiting something. It identifies the purpose of the law, how it is to be interpreted, penalties for failure to adhere to the law and the remedies available to an injured party.

The courts apply a statute to the circumstances in determining whether there has been a breach of the law and then apply the penalties.

Here is an extract from a statute, the Limitation Act 1980.[3]

LIMITATION ACT 1980

(1980 Chapter 58)
An Act to consolidate the Limitation Acts 1939 to 1980
[13 November 1980]

Time limits under Part 1 subject to extension or exclusion under Part II

S 11 Special time limit for actions in respect of personal injuries

(1) This section applies to any action for damages for negligence, nuisance or breach of duty (whether the duty exists by virtue of a contract or of provision made by or under a statute or independently of any contract or any such provision) where the damages claimed by the plaintiff for the negligence, nuisance or breach of duty consist of or include damages in respect of personal injuries to the plaintiff or any other person.

(1A) This section does not apply to any action brought for damages under section 3 of the Protection from Harassment Act 1997.

(2) None of the time limits given in the preceding provisions of this Act shall apply to an action to which this section applies.

(3) An action to which this section applies shall not be brought after the expiration of the period applicable in accordance with subsection (4) or (5) below.

(4) Except where subsection (5) below applies, the period applicable is three years from—

(a) the date on which the cause of action accrued; or

(b) the date of knowledge (if later) of the person injured.

(5) If the person injured dies before the expiration of the period mentioned in subsection (4) above, the period applicable as respects the cause of action surviving for the benefit of his estate by virtue of section 1 of the Law Reform (Miscellaneous Provisions) Act 1934 shall be three years from—

(a) the date of death; or

(b) the date of the personal representative's knowledge; whichever is the later.

The Act above sets out the time within which a person can bring a claim for negligence.

Section 11 (4) (a) and (b) has the effect that a person must bring a claim for negligence within three years from the date on which the cause of action accrued; or the date of knowledge (if later) of the person injured.

Statute and Health Records

Although there is no statute specifically dealing with health records, there are statutes that impact on and apply to them. Examples include:

➤ Freedom of Information Act 2000[4]

➤ Human Rights Act 1998[5]
➤ Data Protection Act 1998[6]
➤ Access to Health Records Act 1990[7]
➤ The Mental Health Act 1983[8]

More detailed information about these Acts can be found in Chapter 13 under the heading 'Patient's right of access to health records'.

Common law (case law)

Where no statute exists, the courts develop law by considering the particular set of circumstances in a case and making a decision. Those decisions become the law – hence the term 'case law'. Important decisions, together with reasons for their decisions, are recorded in Law Reports. These decisions are then followed by the courts when dealing with cases with similar circumstances. If the common law differs from a statute, the statute will overrule the common law.

An example of what a law report looks like is set out below: Bull & Anor v Devon Area Health Authority (1989).[9]

BULL & ANOR V DEVON AREA HEALTH AUTHORITY (1989)

CA (Civ Div) (Slade LJ, Dillon LJ, Mustill LJ) 2/2/89

CLINICAL NEGLIGENCE – CIVIL EVIDENCE – CIVIL PROCEDURE – PERSONAL INJURY

CAUSATION: DUTY OF CARE: BREACH: DOCTORS: SYSTEM FOR SUMMONING: ADEQUATE AND EFFICIENT SYSTEM

Where an expectant mother had been left unattended for an excessive period, health authority's failure to provide and implement an adequate and efficient system for summoning medical practitioners on call held negligent.

Appeal from decision of Tucker J allowing a claim for damages for personal injury, brought by the first plaintiff on her own behalf, and as next friend to her son the second plaintiff, who was the second of uniovular twins born prematurely in the defendant's hospital in March 1970. The first twin was born without complication, but there was a delay of 68 minutes before the second twin was born, due to difficulty in tracing a suitably qualified medical practitioner to assist in the delivery. The second plaintiff suffered brain damage and was severely mentally disabled with spastic quadriplegia. The plaintiffs alleged such injury to have been caused by birth asphyxia resulting from the defendant's negligence. The trial judge held the first plaintiff's claim to be time-barred, but gave judgment for the second plaintiff. On appeal.

HELD: (1) The law allowed a plaintiff under a disability such as this, who was himself without fault, to bring a negligence claim at any time during his life. This being so, his case could not be treated as being prejudiced by the delay, save in that the lapse of time made it harder for him to discharge the onus of proof upon him on the available evidence. (2) (Per Slade LJ) It had not been proven that there was any pulling of the umbilical cord and damage to the placenta after the birth of the first twin, and the trial judge was wrong to conclude that the emergency arose because of the defendant's negligence. (3) (Per Slade LJ) It was not incumbent upon the defendant to ensure that proper assistance was readily available; this was an overstatement of the duty, as to have a registrar constantly available was unrealistic. However, the delays in summoning assistance were so substantial as to place the evidential burden of justifying them on the defendant. (4) Either applying the principle of res ipsa loquitur (per Slade LJ) or on the ordinary civil standard of proof, the defendant had been negligent, in that there was inadequacy or breakdown in the hospital's system for summoning medical assistance, so that the expectant mother was left unattended for an excessive period. (5) There were no grounds for disputing the judge's finding that on the balance of probabilities the delay arising from the defendant's breach of duty was causative of the injury. He had heard the evidence and was entitled to prefer that of one expert, and the Court of Appeal could not retry the case on the transcripts.

Appeal dismissed.

GUIDELINES AND CODES OF PRACTICE

Guidelines, protocols and codes of practice are set down by various bodies; for example, professional bodies, such as the General Medical Council (GMC)[10] and the Nursing and Midwifery Council (NMC),[11] and regulatory bodies, such as the National Institute for Health and Clinical Excellence (NICE)[12] and the Commission for Health Improvement. Guidelines, protocols and codes of practice are also set down at local level issued by, for example, a Trust. These guidelines and protocols provide a safe framework for practice. Whilst they are not legally binding, they are recommended practice. Breaches of them do not usually, in themselves, give rise to civil or criminal liability (except midwives under the NMC *Midwives' Rules*).[13] However, a breach may be evidence of failure to follow the approved practice and it could be argued that such breach constituted negligence.

Furthermore, it must not be forgotten that a failure to adhere to the guidelines or protocols may give rise to repercussions for breach of the professional code of conduct and may constitute a breach of duty of care. The recent case of Cope v Bro Morgannwg NHS Trust 2006[14] illustrates the breach of duty of care for failing to adhere to a policy.

COPE V BRO MORGANNWG NHS TRUST 2006

Mrs Cope contracted MRSA at hospital after a hip replacement operation in February 2001. The infection meant her new hip had to be removed. She took legal action against the Trust that runs the hospital, claiming it had allowed her to contract MRSA by failing to implement its policies and treat the infection appropriately. The hospital accepted it had not followed its own guidelines on infection control in her care.

The case was settled out of court.

COURT STRUCTURE

A breach of the law may give rise to civil or criminal liability. These matters are dealt with by the various courts.

Here is a simplified illustration of court structure (Figure 2.1). Within the court structure there are a variety of branches not illustrated here, such as Family Division, tribunals or inquiries.

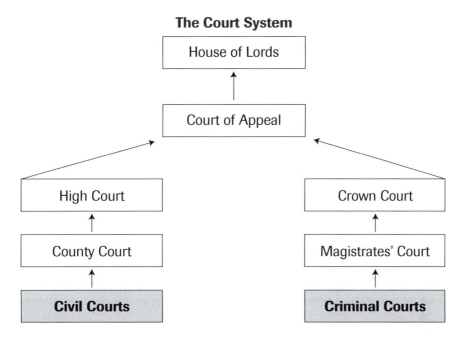

FIGURE 2.1 Court structure

CIVIL LAW

Civil courts deal with civil matters, which can involve money matters, contractual disputes or property issues. They also include negligence, trespass to property or the person, nuisance or breach of statutory duty, amongst other things.

In respect of health professionals, the civil actions that will generally concern them include:

➤ negligence (clinical negligence)
➤ trespass to property or the person
➤ breach of statutory duty.

Where there has been a breach of the civil law then it may give rise to a claim for compensation by the injured party.

NEGLIGENCE

Negligence is also referred to as a breach of the duty of care and occurs when the standard of care falls below the reasonable standard expected. A breakdown of communication either through the records or in some other way may result in an injury to the patient. This may give rise to an action in negligence. If a patient is injured as a result of the negligence of a health professional then the patient may sue for financial compensation. (Compensation is also referred to as 'damages'.)

A person who brings a claim for negligence is called the 'claimant' and the person or organisation being sued is called the 'defendant'. The legal process for bringing a claim is often referred to as 'litigation'.

Duty of care

Record keeping is part of the duty of care owed by health professionals. If the standard of records fall short of what is expected then it may constitute a breach of duty of care. If, as a result, the patient is injured then it may give rise to a claim for compensation.

Donoghue v Stevenson 1932

The leading case of Donoghue v Stevenson[15] changed the law relating to negligence and is commonly referred to as the case of 'the snail in the ginger beer'. A claimant who wishes to bring a claim of negligence has to meet the requirements set out by the House of Lords in this case.[15]

DONOGHUE V STEVENSON 1932

Facts of the case

Mrs Donoghue and her friend were out shopping and stopped for refreshments. Mrs Donoghue's friend treated Mrs Donoghue to a bottle of ginger beer. Her friend treated her not only to the ginger beer, but also to a decomposing snail, which was lurking in the bottom of the bottle. The experience made Mrs Donoghue sick.

Mrs Donoghue sued the café proprietor. The law at this time was based on contractual obligations. The court said Mrs Donoghue had no contract with the café proprietor, as it was her friend who had the contract because it was she who had bought the ginger beer. This was sound legal argument at that time and there was no remedy under the law.

So Mrs Donoghue sued the beer manufacturer. The manufacturer's contract was with the café proprietor, but the manufacturer did not have a contract with Mrs Donoghue and so she lost again.

The matter then went to the Court of Appeal and it was lost on the same principles. There was no contract between Mrs Donoghue, the ginger beer manufacturer or the café proprietor.

Not content with the outcome, Mrs Donoghue took the matter to the House of Lords. (What drove her to do that we will never know!)

The House of Lords said that although there was no contract between Mrs Donoghue and the manufacturer, because Mrs Donoghue was affected by the actions of the manufacturer they must owe her a duty of care.

In this case, the court set out three principles that must be present in order for a person to succeed in a claim for compensation for negligence:

1   the defendant owed the claimant a duty of care; and
2   the defendant breached that duty of care; and
3   the defendant's breach of duty caused the damage to the claimant.

The court will determine as a matter of course that a Trust or health professional will owe a duty of care to their patient. But the patient then has to show that the duty of care was breached and that the breach caused him damage.

What constitutes a breach of duty? The Bolam Principle

The test as to whether health professionals are in breach of their duty of care is whether a responsible body of medical practitioners would have acted in the same way.

A responsible body is judged on the skill of the health professional as outlined in the case of Bolam v Friern Barnet 1957:[16] 'Where a case involves some special skill or competence then the test as to whether there has been negligence or not is based upon the standard of the ordinary skilled man exercising and professing to have that special skill or knowledge.'

Thus the negligence of a health professional, for example, a nurse, will be determined by the standard of the ordinary skilled nurse. This has the effect that the greater the skill, experience and expertise of the health professional, the greater the duty of care. Therefore, a specialist nurse will owe a greater duty than a non-specialist nurse.

Standard of proof

In the civil courts, the standard of proof is 'on the balance of probability'. The court will ask, 'is it more likely than not that a certain set of circumstances occurred?'

In civil cases it is up to the claimant to prove their case.

EXAMPLE OF A CIVIL CASE

A female patient attends hospital complaining of severe stomach cramps. She is examined and tests are carried out. The doctor reassures the patient and says that she has probably eaten something that has upset her stomach and the patient is discharged. Two days later the patient is brought in by ambulance still complaining of severe stomach cramps. On review of the records, the clinical picture was clear that the patient was suffering from an ectopic pregnancy, but the doctor had missed this on the previous occasion. The patient dies in the A&E department before they could take her to theatre.

- Was there a duty of care?
- Did the defendant breach the duty of care? Would a responsible body of medical practitioners have acted in the same way?
- Did the breach of duty of care cause the death of the patient? But for the actions of the doctor, would the patient have died?

If the court were to determine that the responsible body of medical practitioners would have identified the ectopic pregnancy when the patient was first admitted, then the doctor would be in breach of his duty of care. The court will then go on to consider causation – the 'but for' principle. Did the breach of duty result in the patient's death? If the patient had been properly diagnosed and operated on the first day, would she have survived? If the court determines she would have survived if the doctor had properly diagnosed and treated the patient, then the deceased family would succeed in a claim for compensation.

CRIMINAL LAW

Criminal courts deal with criminal matters. Situations giving rise to criminal charges in relation to healthcare may include deliberate harm to a patient (e.g. cases such as Beverly Allitt and Harold Shipman, both of whom killed many of their patients), manslaughter for gross negligence or recklessness, assault and battery, fraud or theft.[17,18]

Deliberate harm caused

BEVERLY ALLITT 1993

Beverly Allitt worked as a nurse at Grantham Hospital. She was suffering from the mental health illness known as Münchausen's syndrome by proxy (a desire to kill or injure others to get attention). In 1993, she was convicted of murdering four children and injuring nine others. She injected babies with high doses of insulin to induce hypoglycaemic seizures and coma. She then attempted to revive them in front of other nurses and the infants' families. She also injected potassium into other children, bringing on convulsions and heart attacks. When she could no longer gain access to such medication she suffocated the infants in her care.

Of course it is rare that a health professional intends to cause harm to a patient. In the usual course of events, the health professional does not intend to cause deliberate harm. Where a patient dies as a result of treatment that was grossly negligent, this can constitute manslaughter. The case of R v Adomako is a prime example.[19]

R V ADOMAKO 1994

This case involved manslaughter by an anaesthetist when, during surgery, the endotracheal tube disconnected and went unnoticed by the anaesthetist. The supply of oxygen to the patient ceased, which led to cardiac arrest and death.

The anaesthetist first became aware that something was wrong when the alarm sounded on the Dinamap machine, which monitors the patient's blood pressure. The evidence was that almost five minutes had elapsed between the disconnection and the alarm sounding. Following the alarm, the anaesthetist responded in various ways by checking the equipment and administering atropine to raise the patient's blood pressure. But at no stage before the cardiac arrest did the anaesthetist check the endotracheal tube connection. The disconnection was not discovered until after resuscitation measures had been commenced.

This situation was considered to be so reckless and grossly negligent that it constituted manslaughter.

Assault and battery

A health professional may commit the criminal offence of assault and battery, for example, by treating a patient without their valid consent.

EXAMPLE OF ASSAULT AND BATTERY

A mother with her son of 8 years and daughter of 7 years attended the dentist. An appointment had been made only for the mother and daughter. Whilst in the waiting room the son went to the bathroom. He was missing for about 15 minutes when his mother became worried. She went to look for him and found him in the dentist chair. Her son had been seen in the corridor by the dentist, who said, 'Come on, chappy, in the chair'. The dentist then proceeded to give him the treatment that was intended for the daughter. The dentist extracted two second molars.

Not only did this constitute a breach of duty of care, but also it was an assault as there was no consent given for the procedure.

Fraud and theft

Other areas where criminal charges may be brought are where there has been fraud or theft. An example of fraud is prescription fraud, which is the illegal acquisition of prescription drugs for personal use or profit. Examples of prescription fraud include stealing a prescription pad to write a prescription for a fictitious patient or altering a prescription in order to increase the quantity of the prescription drug that will be delivered. Theft might include stealing drugs, hospital equipment or a patient's personal belongings.

Standard of proof

In criminal cases, the burden of proof is 'beyond all reasonable doubt'. The jury must be sure of the guilt of the defendant. The standard of proof is higher in criminal cases because somebody's liberty is at stake; therefore, the court has to be sure that an offence has been committed. It is the duty of the prosecution to prove their case against the defendant.

REFERENCES

1 The Mental Health Act 1983.
2 Mental Capacity Act 2005.
3 Limitation Act 1980.
4 Freedom of Information Act 2000.
5 Human Rights Act 1998.
6 Data Protection Act 1998.
7 Access to Health Records Act 1990.
8 The Mental Health Act 1983.
9 Bull & Anor v Devon Area Health Authority [1993] 4 Med. LR 117.
10 www.gmc-uk.org
11 www.nmc-uk.org
12 www.nice.org.uk
13 The Nursing and Midwifery Council. *Midwives' Rules and Standards*. Available at: www.nmc-uk.org/aFrameDisplay.aspx?DocumentID=169 (accessed 10 February 2009).
14 Cope v Bro Morgannwg NHS Trust 2006, unreported. www.brachers.co.uk/_assets/files/Vital%20Signs%20Autumn%202005.pdf
15 Donoghue v Stevenson 1932 AC 562.
16 Bolam v Friern Barnet 1957 2 All ER 118.
17 R v Beverly Allitt 1992. Available at: www.judiciary.gov.uk/docs/judgments_guidance/allitt_061207.pdf
18 R v Harold Shipman 2000. Available at: www.the-shipman-inquiry.org.uk/reports.asp
19 R v Adomako [1995] 1 AC 171; [1994] 3 All ER 79.

CHAPTER 3

Accountability

'Staff were under pressure, but I meant
well. I acted in good faith.'

Over the past few years the ethos in healthcare has changed. Gone are the days when a doctor was put on a pedestal and was not to be challenged; when it was routine to simply say to a patient 'nice to see you, fix you tomorrow'; when health records were marked 'not to be handled by the patient'. Now, of course, we live in a very different environment. Patients are much more aware of their rights. Access to the internet has opened a huge arena for the exchange of information, enabling patients to be more informed.

We have moved very far from the days when the records were not to be handled by the patient. Today, patients have a legal right to access their records and indeed we now have patient-held records.

There are the laws relating to consent. Health professionals have an obligation to obtain the consent of the patient before they can treat them. If health professionals fail to comply with the rules of consent, they are in danger of committing a criminal offence (*see* Chapter 2). For health professionals this means that the law has now become part of their role and is an everyday concern. The complexity of the law does not make this an easy task for them. In a healthcare setting it leaves the health professionals vulnerable. In practice, they go about their daily routines, making decisions about patient care and planning and exercising treatment. It is hoped that the health professional will make the right decisions, that the employer will stand by those decisions and that the courts will uphold those decisions.

Health professionals have concerns about who is responsible when a patient suffers harm. They are often heard in the witness box saying, 'Staff were under pressure, but I meant well. I acted in good faith.' Of course, health professionals do not intend to cause harm; they may have no control over resources or may be ignorant of procedures through lack of training. Can a health professional be held accountable under these circumstances? Yes: these circumstances do not exonerate the health professional from their responsibility. When something goes awry they are accountable.

It is important for health professionals not only to be aware of their legal and professional obligations, but also to put them into perspective – getting the balance right. Often health professionals have an unhealthy fear of the law, causing themselves unnecessary anxiety. This fear is often countered with an unrealistic view that it will never happen to them or that someone else or something else is responsible, 'but not me'. Often a defensive approach is adopted: 'I don't have the time'; 'it's because of financial constraints'; 'it's my manager's responsibility' or 'it's the consultant's responsibility'. The health professional cannot simply pass responsibility like a hot potato. They are accountable for their actions.

My intention is not to alarm the health professional, but to realistically impart the information in a manner whereby a balance may be struck.

The concept of accountability is one which is familiar to all health professionals. It is a word that they all know and use and it forms part of their working-day vocabulary. But how can it be defined?

TASK 3.1

1　Before you read further, try to define 'accountability'.
2　List the areas in which you think you are accountable.

TASK 3.2

Scenario
A nurse is told by a doctor to administer a drug. The nurse is unfamiliar with the drug and says she will check with the pharmacy. The doctor says, 'Don't be impertinent; I have prescribed the drug and you must administer it'. The nurse therefore administers the drug. The patient suffers an adverse reaction because there were contraindications for its use.

Think about this situation and consider:

1   who is accountable?
2   to whom are they accountable?

Read on and we will then review the scenario.

ACCOUNTABILITY IN A LEGAL CONTEXT

In a legal context there is no distinction between responsibility and account-ability. Responsibility can be defined as being accountable for, answerable for and liable to be called to account.

The reality of the situation is that a health professional is, on a personal level, answerable and can be called to account. Once that premise has been accepted, the inevitable and consequent enquiry that must flow from that is how and to whom is that accountability discharged? How far the health professional can be held accountable for their actions is not within the ambit of this book.

The discharge of the duty is debated by, and lies with, the courts. The law, by its nature, is reactive and is invoked after the event. It is only when a real case is presented that the judges will deliberate and deliver judgment. It follows then that issues are debated with the benefit of hindsight. Thus, we cannot go to the courts with hypothetical questions or scenarios; for example, 'If I do it in particular way, will I be in trouble?' The usual sequence is that something will have happened to trigger an investigation. This will raise the question of accountability. When the health professional appears before the court his acts or omissions will be weighed up and judgment will be delivered. The practical effect is that health professionals make decisions about patient care and it is hoped that the courts will ultimately support them.

Now that we've put accountability into its legal context the next question is: to whom is the health professional accountable?

TASK 3.3

■   To whom are you accountable?

List your answers.

THE FOUR AREAS OF ACCOUNTABILITY

There is not just one single individual or body to whom the health professional is accountable; in fact, there are four:

➤ society
➤ patient
➤ employer
➤ professional body.

Having established that the health professional can be accountable in four quite distinct respects, we need next to examine how accountability impacts in practice.

Society

Health professionals are accountable to society for issues that are in the public interest. Society dictates the kind of behaviour they will and will not accept. If someone is murdered, society says this is wrong and the murderer must be punished. Society's view is then enshrined in criminal law. We have seen manslaughter charges brought against schoolteachers where a child has died on a school trip. These charges are brought because the teachers have not lived up to the trust that society imposes. It will be argued that the individual has fallen short of what society accepts and demands of someone in that position. If the person is found guilty, they face a penalty. As society's values change then the law may also change to reflect these changes. For example, suicide used to be considered a crime, but is no longer; the law has changed to reflect this.

When dealing with accountability to society the discharge of such accountability rests with the criminal court. This court acts in the public interest.

Criminal proceedings are brought against an individual. It is personal. The criminal court punishes the individual guilty of an offence. It is not possible for the individual to be indemnified by the employer or defence union. The health professional's boss is not going to say, 'Don't worry, I'll serve your sentence for you'!

In a case involving the Ford motor company, an employee died from falling into a vat of paint and drowning. The director was found guilty and personally fined £5000. The court made it clear this was to be paid by the director himself and not the company. The reason for this is that it is personal, and the individual found guilty of an offence cannot be indemnified. They will be punished.

The kinds of sanctions that may be imposed by the criminal courts include:
➤ custodial sentence (imprisonment)
➤ a fine
➤ community-based sentences.

Any criminal conviction of a health professional is reported to the professional body concerned. (*See* Chapter 2 where we have already taken a brief look at the criminal process.)

Patient

Health professionals are accountable to the patient or client. The discharge of accountability rests with the civil courts. Civil law is not about punishment, unlike the criminal process. If a patient is injured as a result of negligent treatment, the patient may seek financial compensation through the civil courts. The purpose of the patient suing for compensation is to put them back into the position they would have been in financially if the incident had not occurred.

EXAMPLE OF BEING ACCOUNTABLE TO A PATIENT OR CLIENT

A patient attends hospital as a day patient for the removal of a polyp under general anaesthetic. Due to an error with the records the patient is added to the wrong theatre list and, instead of carrying out the removal of the polyp, the patient's leg is amputated by mistake. The patient sues for compensation for financial loss. Had the correct procedure been carried out the patient would have had the polyp removed and then been discharged that day. He would have returned to work and resumed his usual daily life. However, now the patient's condition is such that he has to stay in hospital, cannot return to work (so he's lost his income), he will require care at home, equipment and further treatment, which he will now have to pay for. The damages the patient claims are to recompense him for this financial loss. There will also be some recompense for pain and suffering.

The value of such claims will vary as it is based on the loss endured by the individual. The same circumstances may arise with two patients but one claim may be valued at £5000 whereas the other might be valued at £5 million. The difference is that if the first patient was unemployed at the time of the incident and never likely to work in any event then there is no claim for loss of earnings. However, the second patient may be a professional footballer at the peak of his career and therefore the loss of earnings could be very substantial.

Employer

If a patient has been injured constituting negligence, for example, as a result of poor records, the patient may sue for compensation. Who does the patient sue, the individual health professional or the Trust?

Some employers accept liability for negligent acts and/or omissions by their employees. This is known as vicarious liability. Such cover does not normally extend to activities undertaken outside the health professional's employment. Independent practice would not normally be covered by vicarious liability.

If a health professional is self-employed or works in the private health sector, it is the individual health professional's responsibility to establish their insurance status and take appropriate action. In situations where employers do not accept vicarious liability, then it is recommended that health professionals should obtain adequate professional indemnity insurance. If a health professional is unable to secure professional indemnity insurance, they will need to demonstrate that all their clients/patients are fully informed of this fact and the implications this might have in the event of a claim for professional negligence.

Where the employer is vicariously liable for the employee they are liable for their acts and omissions. It does not matter whether the employee is full-time, part-time, temporary or agency staff, they will be considered as acting as an agent for the Trust. In practical terms, this means the Trust is responsible for the actions of their employees. It therefore follows that although the individual health professional may have been negligent, the employer will meet any claim for compensation. Thus the health professionals concerned in the incident do not themselves have to pay the compensation.

Whilst there is nothing in law preventing the patient suing the individual health professional, the patient will usually choose to sue the Trust rather than the individual. This is because the Trust is more likely to have the financial resources to pay the compensation. There is no point in suing a man of straw (someone with no money).

There are, however, exceptions to this. In certain circumstances, the Trust may recoup the compensation they have paid from the individuals concerned in the incident. However, this should only be pursued in exceptional circumstances. Exceptional circumstances are likely to include causing deliberate harm, such as in the Beverly Allitt case.[1] However, the Nursing and Midwifery Council (NMC)[2] make it clear that where a nurse prescribes outside her powers then the Trust may not stand by her. Therefore, it is recommended that health professionals have indemnity insurance in place.

The Trust sought to recover from Beverly Allitt the compensation paid out to her victims. In reality, of course, the Trust is unlikely to recover the compensation from her because she is in prison, has no income and is therefore unlikely to have the resources to pay back the money.

The reason a Trust may seek to recover such compensation is public perception. They do not want the public to that think they are condoning this kind of behaviour. They will also wish to recoup public money.

Notwithstanding that it is the Trust, not the individual, that will be sued, and that it is the Trust that will pay out the compensation, this does not exonerate the health professional and they are still accountable to their employer.

The employer may be unhappy about what has happened and may look into the matter. The employer will be concerned with the contract of employment and whether there has been any breach of that contract and whether the employee has acted outside their job description.

EXAMPLE OF A HEALTH PROFESSIONAL WORKING OUTSIDE THEIR JOB DESCRIPTION

A district nurse who for many years worked in community care took up a new post in the A&E Department. The standard job description was that only a doctor could suture hands and face. A patient was admitted whose face required suturing. The nurse considered herself far more experienced than the junior doctors, so she did suture the patient's face. It all went wrong and the patient was left with scarring that could have been avoided. The employer considered that the nurse was in breach of her contract of employment because the job description was clear: it prohibited her from suturing a patient's face. The employer dismissed the nurse from employment.

It is implied in a contract of employment that an employee will obey reasonable instructions of the employer and that the employee will use all their care and skill in carrying out their duties. As an employee, the health professional cannot embark on a 'frolic of their own'. They are answerable to the employer and it is the responsibility of the employer to look at the circumstances of breach of contract and address it.

The kinds of sanctions the employer can invoke are:
➤ grievance procedure
➤ disciplinary procedure.

This could lead to:
➤ warning
➤ demotion
➤ suspension
➤ dismissal.

Health professionals are answerable to their employer, which may result in disciplinary action with sanctions. The ultimate sanction is, of course, dismissal.

Professional body

Professional bodies are the organisations that regulate health professionals. Their primary aim is to protect the public. This is achieved by setting and maintaining standards of education, training, conduct and performance that the public is entitled to expect. These are usually set out in their codes of conduct. It is the responsibility of the health professionals to be familiar with their duties and codes of conduct.

The professional body will look at whether the health professional is competent to practise, whether they are safe, whether they have maintained professional standards and so on.

Information about a health professional may be received by the professional body from a number of sources. Anyone has the right to make a complaint. If there is a criminal conviction it will be reported to the professional body. Non-criminal misconduct may also be reported. A health professional may be reported by a judge following a civil court hearing. Reports may also be received from the police, a patient or their family, the health professional's employer, managers, colleagues and other health professionals. The professional body will then investigate the matter and this may result in a hearing before a conduct and competence committee to decide the case.

There are many regulatory bodies governing healthcare. They include, for example:

➤ Nursing and Midwifery Council (NMC)[2]
➤ General Medical Council (GMC)[3]
➤ General Dental Council (GDC)[4]
➤ General Chiropractic Council (GCC)[5]
➤ General Optical Council (GOC)[6]
➤ Royal Pharmaceutical Society of Great Britain (RPSGB).[7]

These professional bodies will be concerned with issues surrounding fitness to practise and the health professional's suitability to be on the register without restrictions. They will consider whether the health professional's fitness to practise is impaired. Issues that can impair this include:

➤ **Lack of competence**; for example:
  — persistent lack of ability in correctly and/or appropriately calculating, administering and recording the administration or disposal of medicines
  — persistent lack of ability in properly identifying care needs and, accordingly
  — planning and delivering appropriate care.
➤ **Physical or mental ill health**; for example:
  — alcohol or drug dependence
  — untreated serious mental illness.
➤ **Misconduct**; for example:
  — physical or verbal abuse
  — theft
  — deliberate failure to deliver adequate care
  — deliberate failure to keep proper records.
➤ **A finding by any other health or social care regulator or licensing body** that a registrant's fitness to practise is impaired.
➤ **A conviction or caution** (including a finding of guilty by a court martial); for example:
  — theft
  — fraud or other dishonest activities
  — violence
  — sexual offences

— accessing or downloading child pornography or other illegal material from the internet
— illegally dealing in or importing drugs.

➤ **Fraudulent or incorrect entry in the professional register.**

Sanctions that can be imposed by a professional body

There are sanctions that can be imposed by the professional bodies. The purpose of such sanctions is not to punish the health professional but to protect the public.

The types of sanctions that can be imposed include:

➤ a 'conditions of practice' order; for example, they may impose conditions the health professional must comply with, such as requiring him to undertake training or work with supervision

➤ a caution order

➤ a suspension order

➤ a striking-off order.

Private activities

Health professionals also need to be aware that regulatory bodies can look at the private activities of the health professional to assess whether they are fit to practise.

The NMC guidelines state:

> You must behave in a way that upholds the reputation of the professions.[8]

Behaviour that compromises this reputation may call your registration into question even if is not directly connected to your professional practice.

An example of sanctions in action was a health professional who was removed from the register for soliciting a woman for prostitution.

Standard of record keeping

A health professional can be called into question as to their fitness to practise for failing to adequately maintain a patient's health records.

In a recent case, a registered nurse was charged by the NMC for failing to make records of immunisations administered to patients. The NMC issued a caution as to future conduct of this nurse.

There are many examples where poor records have led to sanctions, including striking-off being imposed by the professional bodies.

The NMC's *The Code*[9] states that a health professional must keep clear and accurate records. If the health professional fails to do so they will be held accountable. The NMC also sets out guidance for record keeping, which all health professionals will find useful. The records are explored in more detail in Chapters 5–11.

Accountability

The healthcare professional can be called to account in all four areas of accountability, which means that in effect they can be tried four times. The case of Beverly Allitt is an illustration of this.[1]

THE ACCOUNTABILITY OF BEVERLY ALLITT

Society – Beverly Allitt was accountable to society. She was considered to have failed society by committing the criminal offences of killing and injuring children. For this she was prosecuted in the criminal courts and a custodial sentence was imposed.

Patient – Beverly Allitt was accountable to the patients. The parents of the deceased and injured children brought civil claims for compensation. The Trust paid out the compensation.

Employer – Her employers pursued disciplinary proceedings against her and she was dismissed from her employment.

Professional Body – The professional body removed her from the register.

Where a health professional is not a member of a professional body (e.g. a healthcare assistant), they should still follow professional standards and they will still be called to account in the other areas of accountability.

It is important for health professionals to appreciate that the four areas of accountability are separate and distinct. Where, for example, due to lack of resources, the Trust condones or turns a blind eye to the carrying out of duties that are beyond the skill of the health professional, the Trust may decide to take no disciplinary action. However, the Trust cannot protect the health professional from the other areas of accountability. So if the patient was harmed, despite the Trust having turned a blind eye, the patient can still sue, criminal charges can be brought against the health professionals and the professional body can step in. It is no defence for the health professional to say that the Trust knew about it. The health professional will still be held accountable for their actions.

It does not necessarily follow that if an employer dismisses the health professional, the professional body will strike a health professional from the register. Nor does it necessarily follow that if the professional body strikes someone from the register they will be dismissed from their employment. However, in the latter circumstances, the health professional concerned would lose their registered position.

REVIEW OF THE SCENARIO (*SEE* TASK 3.2)

A nurse is told by a doctor to administer a drug. The nurse is unfamiliar with the drug and says she will check with the pharmacy. The doctor says, 'Don't be impertinent; I have prescribed the drug and you must administer it'. The nurse therefore administers the drug. The patient suffers an adverse reaction because there were contraindications for its use.

1 Who is accountable?
  Answer – Both the doctor and the nurse will be accountable.

2 To whom are they accountable?
  Answer – they are accountable to the patient who may bring a claim for harm suffered, the employer and the professional body.

LEGAL AND PROFESSIONAL OBLIGATIONS

Here is a brief checklist of legal and professional obligations that impact on health professionals:
➤ statute
➤ common law
➤ guidelines
➤ accountability
  — society
  — patient
  — employer
  — professional body.

In order to be responsible, it is necessary for the health professional to have knowledge of the law and to remember that ignorance of the law is no defence.

REFERENCES

1 R v Beverly Allitt 1992. Available at: www.judiciary.gov.uk/docs/judgments_guidance/allitt_061207.pdf
2 www.nmc-uk.org
3 www.gmc-uk.org
4 www.gdc-uk.org
5 www.gcc-uk.org
6 www.optical.org
7 www.rpsgb.org.uk
8 Nursing and Midwifery Council. *The Code*. Standards of conduct, performance and ethics for nurses and midwives code of professional conduct 2008. Available at: www.nmc-uk.org/aFrameDisplay.aspx?DocumentID=3954
9 Nursing and Midwifery Council. *The Code*. Available at: www.nmc-uk.org/aSection.aspx?SectionID=45 (accessed 9 February 2009).

CHAPTER 4

Will the records stand up to legal scrutiny?

*'It was poor documentation that resulted in
the unnecessary death of this patient.'*

CASE STUDY

This is a real case and illustrates many of the issues covered in this book
including:

➤ record keeping
➤ breakdown of communication
➤ inconsistencies between the records and other documents
➤ the court's view of the records
➤ accountability of the health professionals.

Facts of the case

This case involved an elderly gentleman (the patient) who had suffered
intermittently from psoriasis for many years and from time to time it would
flare up. He was otherwise fit and mobile. On this occasion he had a flare up
on the soles of his feet and a localised rash in the groin area.

He was regularly visited at home by a podiatrist who advised, 'Why don't
you go and see a consultant dermatologist who will sort this rash out for you?'
The patient saw the consultant dermatologist on a private basis. The consultant diagnosed psoriasis and gave the patient a prescription for non-steroidal

anti-inflammatory cream. The consultant said, 'If that doesn't work I will admit you into hospital and carry out some tests and I will sort the rash out for you once and for all'.

The patient applied the non-steroidal anti-inflammatory cream, but it exacerbated the rash, which became red. So the patient telephoned the GP who said, 'Stop using the cream and go back and see the consultant'. The patient saw the consultant again on a private basis and the consultant made arrangements for the patient to be admitted into hospital under the NHS. The patient was admitted several weeks later and was under the care of the same consultant he had seen on a private basis.

However, on admission of the patient the consultant was away on a training course and would be away for the next seven days. There was no handover by the consultant of this patient and the private notes were not made available to the NHS hospital. The patient was admitted by an SHO who wrote in the clinical records, 'Admitted with psoriasis'. The SHO also wrote in the clinical records, 'Allergy to penicillin' but did not record this allergy to penicillin on the drug chart or in the designated box on the front of the records.

For the first week the consultant was away on the course and so did not see the patient. For the first four days the nursing staff applied non-steroidal anti-inflammatory creams. On about day four the rash had reddened and a blister had appeared in the groin area. A nurse had noticed this blister and telephoned the SHO to seek advice as to how she should treat the patient. She told the SHO, 'A blister has appeared, what do I do?'

The SHO replied, 'Don't ask me. I have been on this ward for only three weeks; I know nothing about dermatology'.

The nurse then telephoned another doctor. She repeated what she had said to the SHO: 'A blister has appeared, what do I do?'

The doctor said, 'I'm really not sure what to prescribe for this patient'.

So the nurse then telephoned the ward sister to ask for advice. Once more she said, 'A blister has appeared, what do I do?'

Over the telephone, without seeing the patient, the ward sister prescribed Dermovate. (Dermovate is an extremely potent substance and is a prescription only medicine for good reason – because of its potency.)

There were several problems at this point: (i) the ward sister did not have prescribing powers so was not suitably qualified to prescribe this medication; (ii) there were contraindications for the use of Dermovate with this patient; for example, it should not be used in the folds of the skin, so it was inappropriate to use in the groin area; and (iii) there were other contraindications – Dermovate is known to cause blistering.

For whatever reasons, possibly because the nursing sister did not have prescribing powers or she had given the advice over the telephone and did not have the records to hand, she omitted to write up the prescription on the drug chart.

The nurse made good entries in the record about the patient's condition, the detail of the telephone calls and advice she had been given by the doctors and the ward sister. She also made entries in the nursing records that Dermovate was being applied.

The Dermovate exacerbated the patient's condition. By day seven the rash in the groin area had worsened and was by then quite a bullous rash.

On day seven the consultant returned from his course and was faced with a patient with a bullous rash. He had the clinical records to hand but no nursing records, and there was nothing recorded on the drug chart. The consultant was therefore ignorant of the fact that Dermovate was being applied and that this could have been the cause of the bullous rash.

On the basis of the clinical picture the consultant made a diagnosis and entered it in the record: 'pemphigoid?' Pemphigoid is a significant skin condition, but it is not immediately life threatening. It is easy to test for, to diagnose then treat, or to rule out. However, no tests were carried out and no swabs or skin biopsies were taken. But on the basis of the clinical picture the consultant prescribed a high dose steroid, 80 mg.

The following day the patient was catheterised. Over the following few days the catheter fell out. According to the records it had been pulled out by a nurse during bathing on at least two occasions, and then reinserted. The patient's condition deteriorated so he was prescribed penicillin!

The patient then developed an all-over rash – this, in a patient who is already suffering from a skin condition. The following day the error was realised and the penicillin was withdrawn.

However, the patient's condition continued to deteriorate. On day 12 the patient was reviewed by the consultant who considered that his condition was either 'pemphigoid or toxic epidermal necrolysis (TEN)' and made this entry in the records.

TEN is a life-threatening skin condition. It is a rare condition that affects the whole body where blisters occur and the epidermis peels off in large sheets. Widespread areas of erosion, including all mucous membranes (eyes, mouth, genitalia), occur within 24–72 hours, and the patient usually becomes gravely ill. Affected areas of skin often resemble second-degree burns. Death is caused by fluid and electrolyte imbalance and multiorgan sequelae (e.g. pneumonia, gastrointestinal bleeding, glomerulonephritis, hepatitis, infection). A patient with TEN is usually treated as a burns patient, transferred to a burns unit, barrier nursed and so on. However, this patient did not have these classic signs; he had a localised rash in the groin area and neither was he treated as if he had TEN (i.e. transferred to burns unit, etc.).

TEN is a drug-induced condition and there are only a handful of known drugs that cause it. But there was nothing they had given this patient – at least there was nothing recorded on the drug chart – that could have caused TEN. On the basis of the differential diagnosis of pemphigoid or TEN the consultant increased the steroid dosage to 100 mg.

By day 14 the patient's condition had deteriorated further and the rash had not improved. The patient was reviewed by the consultant, who considered that if it had been TEN or pemphigoid, then the steroid would have had some effect. So the plan was to 'withdraw steroid by tapering over the following four days'. The consultant made this entry in the records.

That day a nurse transposed this information from the clinical records into the nursing records as 'withdraw steroid'. Someone then drew a line through the steroid prescription on the drug chart, which resulted in the steroid being withdrawn abruptly. The next day the patient had some coffee-ground vomit. The patient went into shock and died the following day.

This patient was admitted with nothing more than a localised rash of psoriasis, but within two weeks he had died.

The complaints process

There were many issues in this case, including poor handing of the complaints process.

The family were with the patient when he had a rigor. They asked to see the nursing sister to enquire as to his condition and planned care, etc. One of them asked, 'Why is my father shaking?' The response from the nursing sister was, 'Don't worry about that, he's on a vibrating bed'! This undermined the intelligence of the family and alarm bells started ringing.

When the patient died the family wanted to understand what had happened. The explanation given by the nursing sister was, 'He was old; he was going to die anyway'. Such an insensitive comment and lack of openness served only to compound the situation.

It is reasonable for the family to enquire about what has happened. They cannot put closure on it until they have understood the circumstances. They often carry the guilt. In this case, the patient's wife was beside herself. 'I should never have let him go into hospital; it was only a rash,' she said. In the absence of a reasonable explanation they commenced the formal complaint process.

When a complaint is made it is normal procedure for the Trust to ask those involved in the patient's care to provide a statement explaining the details of their involvement. Once this has been gathered the complaints department usually send a letter to the family, signed by the chief executive, giving an explanation of the events. However, in this case, the consultant was not very helpful to the complaints department and refused to be drawn on the issues, saying, 'I refuse to explain the use of a high-dose steroid to these lay people!' This approach made it difficult for the complaints department to provide a reasonable response to the family. Neither did the Trust provide the family with the records despite their request.

In the absence of an explanation, the family requested the next step, which was to have a round table meeting. At the meeting the consultant said, 'I am a very busy man; you have five minutes of my time'. When the family asked a question, the response was, 'I can't answer that; I don't have the records'. So the meeting was a waste of time and the family still had no explanation of what had happened. Their only recourse then was to go to the law.

The process of litigation

During the first stages of litigation there is a process called the 'pre-action protocol for the resolution of clinical disputes'. The purpose of this process is to encourage the parties to resolve the matter at an early stage without the need for court proceedings.

The first step is for the patient's lawyer to investigate the case. The Trust will also carry out its own investigation. The investigation involves obtaining the records and, usually, expert evidence. The expert evidence should be independent. A letter of claim is sent to the Trust setting out the details, the allegations and any proposal for financial settlement.

In the case above, following the investigation, the family had an understanding of what had happened and were ready to put closure on it. They wanted to settle the matter and agreed to do so at an undervalue. The claim was worth in the region of £25 000 and in order to encourage a swift settlement they agreed to accept £15 000.

There were obvious problems with the care of the patient. It was alleged that the Trust had been negligent in its treatment of the patient and had caused his death. A letter of claim was sent to the Trust setting this out and offering to settle the claim at an undervalue. However, the Trust defended the action.

The evidence

The death certificate recorded cause of death as a 'perforated stomach ulcer' and 'TEN'.

There was no evidence that this patient had a perforated stomach ulcer. There was no history; there was nothing noted in the records. If there was a stomach ulcer it had not been identified or treated.

There was no evidence the patient died from TEN. He did not have the classic signs of TEN. The patient's symptoms were not consistent with such a diagnosis in that he had only a localised rash. As previously stated, it is in any event a drug-induced condition and there was nothing they had given the patient that would have caused TEN.

It was difficult though to determine what had caused the patient's death. There were very few tests carried out and no swabs or skin biopsies had been taken. The last blood test was taken on day 11 of his admission, which showed a systemic infection. On balance the claimant's expert thought it more likely that the cause of death was septicaemia. The most common cause of hospital-acquired infection, which can result in septicaemia, is through catheterisation. The patient had been catheterised and there had been problems with the catheter falling out and being reinserted. This had been compounded by the fact that the patient was on a high-dose steroid, which had compromised his immune system. No post-mortem had been carried out.

The Trust, through their legal representatives, defended the claim. They said, 'The patient was admitted with a life-threatening condition'. Well, the records were clear and unambiguous. The SHO had recorded that the patient was admitted with psoriasis, and this is not life threatening. The Trust said, 'The SHO made an error in the records'. But if the patient had been admitted with a life-threatening condition, according to the records the patient was treated inappropriately. He was not treated as if he had such a condition. All they did for the first three to four days was to apply non-steroidal anti-inflammatory creams, which is hardly the treatment for patient who has a life-threatening condition.

The Trust said, 'Well then, it was on day seven that he had a life-threatening condition. This was when a diagnosis of TEN was made and that was why a high-dose steroid was commenced'. But the records state 'pemphigoid?' Whilst pemphigoid is a significant skin condition, it is not immediately life threatening and tests could have established this or ruled it out. There is no mention of TEN in the records on day seven. The Trust said, 'The consultant wrote pemphigoid in the records, but what he really had in the back of his mind was TEN'!

The claimants were not convinced. TEN is a very rare condition. If the consultant really believed the patient had TEN he would have been calling students for miles around to come and have a look, let alone forgetting to write it in the records. More importantly, how are the staff supposed to know what they are treating if the information is in someone's head and not in the records? The Trust continued to defend the action and it proceeded to full trial.

The court's view

The matter took another four years to come to trial. One of the reasons it took so long was the constant changing of the chronology of events. Each time the chronology changed, the evidence had to be reviewed by the experts.

In respect of the documentation, at the trial the court was faced with this scenario:
- failure to provide the NHS hospital with the private health records, resulting in the breakdown of communication about the patient's condition on admission
- error in the admission notes made by the SHO about the patient's condition on admission
- failure by the SHO to record the allergy to penicillin in the designated box on the front of the records and on the drug chart, resulting in the erroneous administering of penicillin
- failure by the nursing sister in prescribing Dermovate without prescribing powers and failing to record it on the drug chart, resulting in a breakdown of communication
- failure by the consultant to have the nursing records to hand during the ward round, resulting in a breakdown of communication
- failure by the consultant to record the diagnosis of TEN on day seven, resulting in the staff not knowing what they were treating

➤ failure by nursing staff incorrectly transposing information from the clinical records into the nursing records relating to the withdrawal of the steroid and someone drawing a line through the prescription of the steroid on the drug chart, resulting in the abrupt withdrawal of the steroid causing the patient to go into shock

➤ inconsistencies between what the SHO said in evidence and what the records stated

➤ inconsistencies between what the consultant said in evidence and what was stated in the records.

Faced with this scenario of errors in the records and inconsistencies between the records and what was said in evidence, the court suggested that the lack of care in record keeping extended to the lack of care of the patient.

The court found in favour of the claimant's family, notwithstanding the fact that it was not certain how or why this patient had died.

What angered the court was the poor documentation that had resulted in the breakdown of communication. The records were inaccurate; there was a failure to record crucial information and as a result inappropriate treatment was commenced. More importantly, it was the poor documentation that had resulted in the unnecessary death of this patient.

Disclosure

Anything you write has the potential to become a legal document. This includes the health records and the complaints file, including all of the documents accumulated through the internal enquiry. In this case, all documents, including the faxes passing between the consultant and the complaints manager, post-it notes, etc., were disclosed.

What lessons were learnt

In this case, there was a failure by the Trust to acknowledge that there was a problem with the documentation and the management of the patient. Good risk management is asking 'what if' and putting procedures in place to avoid the risk from happening. If risk management results from an incident or an audit this is not good management. But, of course, once a problem has been identified then it must be addressed to prevent its happening again.

Consequences for the health professionals

The court in this case enquired whether changes had been made during the intervening four years and whether anyone had been held accountable. Neither had been addressed by the Trust and the court took the step of reporting the consultant and the nursing sister to their professional bodies where misconduct hearings took place.

CHAPTER 5

Good practice for health records

*'I am sorry the patient died, but I didn't
have time to write the records.'*

This chapter on health records sets out a guide for good practice. It is important for health professionals to be familiar with the policies and guidance about records provided by their professional bodies and also policies and guidelines set down at a local level. The good practice guide set out in this chapter should be read alongside these professional and local guidelines. Where there is a conflict between them, the professional and local policies should be followed, unless there is good reason to depart from them. Remember, the health professional will be accountable for their records and the decisions made.

Good record keeping is an essential tool for managing risks. Health professionals have a legal and professional obligation to maintain a reasonable standard of records. It could be argued that a health professional has not discharged their duty of care if the records have not been maintained.

Record keeping is an integral part of patient care and records should provide a clear, accurate account of that care. Good record keeping helps to protect the welfare of patients.

Midwives must ensure that they are aware of and comply with the requirements set out in the NMC's *Midwives' Rules and Standards*[1] that relate to the maintenance and retention of records.

Health professionals working with patients who are subject to mental health legislation must ensure they have a thorough working knowledge of the statutory powers that apply to their particular area of practice. When making entries in records for these patients, they must comply as appropriate with the guidance given by the Mental Health Act Commission for England and Wales,[2] the Mental Welfare Commission for Scotland[3] or the Mental Health Commission for Northern Ireland.[4]

There are a number of key principles that underpin good records and record keeping. Some of these relate to the content and style of the record in addition to the legal issues that a health professional should be aware of and take into account in record-keeping practice.

This guide to record keeping cannot cover every situation or provide the answer to every question or issue that could arise. However, it will assist health professionals by enabling them to apply its principles to any situation. It will help them to think through some of the issues involved and to exercise their professional judgment. Furthermore, it will help them to reflect upon and develop their current record-keeping practice, and therefore it will benefit patients. The principles apply across all care settings and relate to both written and electronic records.

When making entries in the records, health professionals should bear in mind how much their colleagues will rely on these records. Good communication is therefore essential.

Good record keeping promotes:
➤ high standards of patient care
➤ continuity of care
➤ better communication and dissemination of information between members of the inter-professional healthcare team
➤ an accurate account of treatment and care planning and delivery
➤ the ability to detect problems, such as changes in the patient's condition, at an early stage.

Good record keeping is a mark of the skilled and safe practitioner, whilst careless or incomplete record keeping often highlights wider problems with the individual's practice. Poor records reflect poor patient care.

Poor record keeping:
➤ undermines patient care
➤ makes health professionals vulnerable to legal and professional problems

➤ increases workloads
➤ reflects a poor standard of professional practice.

Jennifer Doohan of the Royal College of Nursing, East Midlands, stated at a multidisciplinary meeting in August 2006 regarding the records that, '. . . poor records and record keeping contribute significantly to risks in delivering healthcare, and feedback from Coroners' reports and Health Service Commissioners' comments stressed the need for clear, contemporaneous record keeping to prevent mistakes . . .'[5]

The purpose of the health records is to support high standards of patient care. In addition, the records may also be used for:
➤ evidence-based clinical practice
➤ supporting administrative and managerial decision making
➤ meeting the legal requirements under, for example, the Data Protection Act
➤ assisting clinical and other audits
➤ supporting auditing and clinical governance
➤ supporting improvements for clinical effectiveness
➤ supporting patient choice and control over treatment services
➤ responding to complaints
➤ evidence in claims, complaints, inquests, inquiries and disciplinary hearings and other legal proceedings
➤ refreshing the memory in any legal proceedings.

Care is shared between a number of health professionals and the records should provide an effective means of communication. If a health professional failed to maintain adequate records, and thus did not communicate something to a colleague who then acted in a way that was detrimental to the patient, this would give rise to a legal claim and would also constitute professional misconduct. In making a record, the health professional should also be aware of the reliance that their professional colleagues will have upon it. Therefore, good communication is essential.

Patient records are sometimes called in evidence in order to investigate a complaint, a legal claim, for criminal proceedings or by the professional bodies' Fitness to Practise Committees. The approach to record keeping that courts of law adopt is, 'if it is not recorded, it has not been done, has not been considered or was not said'.

Health professionals should bear in mind that their records will at some time be seen and scrutinised by others. In addition to being shared with other healthcare providers, they will be looked at by the patients, the courts in civil or criminal proceedings or a Coroner's court, for research, teaching or auditing. They will be seen by managers through the complaints process. Remember, records may be relied upon in court not only in matters where the writer is called into question, but also in matters generally involving a patient.

EXAMPLE SITUATION

A patient is recovering from surgery for a hip operation following a fall. He has been discharged and is being looked after at home by district nurses and carers. The district nurse suspects that his wound is infected and asks the General Practitioner (GP) to visit the patient. The GP tells the district nurse he will do so, but does not actually visit. The following day the district nurse considers that the patient has deteriorated and makes a further call to the GP. The GP does not consider it necessary to attend the patient. The district nurse is very concerned about the patient's condition so telephones for an ambulance and the patient is taken to the A&E department. On admission the patient is very poorly and dies shortly afterwards. The family complain that the GP ought to have visited the patient the day before and that, had the GP done so, the patient would have been sent to hospital sooner and would not have died. They initiate a claim for compensation through the civil courts. In addition, the case goes before the Coroner's court.

In these circumstances, the allegations are potentially against the GP, but in order for the court to reach a decision on the success or otherwise of a claim the court will wish to see the whole picture. What was the patient's condition before he was discharged following surgery? What was the patient's condition whilst he was under the community care? What was the patient's condition on admission to A&E?

In order to see the whole picture the court will want to see all the records relating to these issues and hear evidence from the writers of all those records. So the records of the district nurse, the A&E records, and the hospital records of the surgery and care prior to discharge, will all be reviewed by the lawyers and courts. The records then will be looked at for the purpose of investigating the complaint and for the legal claim. The health professionals responsible for the entries may be required to give evidence. Will those records stand up to legal scrutiny?

Through the case study in Chapter 4, I have already highlighted the importance of good record keeping and the consequences of getting it wrong. The best practice guidelines cannot cover every eventuality or entry that a health professional may write, but the principles should be adopted and then applied to their areas of practice.

The health professionals that follow these best practice guidelines will promote consistency and will improve and maintain standards that are essential for patient care and risk management.

THE PURPOSE OF HEALTH RECORDS

Thinking about the purpose of maintaining records will help the health professional to include the appropriate level of detail, content and form, and to write more clearly and accurately.

TASK 5.1

Why do you keep records?
- List the reasons why you think the records are maintained

The primary purpose for health records is to facilitate the care, treatment and support of the patient. Record keeping is a fundamental part of patient care. If a situation were to arise where the health professional was responsible for the total delivery of care and the case load was of such a size that every detail relating to each patient could be remembered in its entirety, then maybe there would not be a need for record keeping. The reality, of course, is very different. As previously mentioned, care is shared between a number of health professionals. Patient records provide health professionals with a means to communicate – they ensure continuity of care, provide a history and act as an aide-memoire. The records should be written in such a way that any health professional could pick up those records and continue with patient care, almost unnoticed from the patient's point of view. Care will be provided by highly qualified, experienced staff that may be very familiar with the patient. However, the patient will also be seen by many health professionals, including students, agency staff, new staff, those less familiar with the patient, health professionals in the community care, acute care and those in other disciplines, such as social services. The records will be relied upon by all of those caring for the patient and they will need to grasp the issues very quickly. They need to be able to pick up those records and hit the ground running. Therefore records should be written in a manner that ensures good communication to enable continuity of care.

A common reason given by health professionals as to why they keep records is 'to cover my back'. This defensive approach to record keeping is inappropriate and as a result often moves away from the primary purpose of facilitating treatment, care and support of the patient. It can have an adverse effect as these defensive records tend to concentrate on the wrong issues and so move away from their real purpose; thus resulting in a breakdown of communication and compromising patient care.

EXAMPLE OF DEFENSIVE RECORD KEEPING

One set of records reads along the lines of:

> 'Patient wants a bar of chocolate' . . . 'patient wants to telephone her mother' . . . 'patient wants to go outside and have a cigarette' . . . 'patient gave me a dirty look on the stairs witnessed by Sandra'.

There were no other entries in the records. Why do you think the records were written in this way?

When the health professional was asked this question the response was 'because this patient was trouble'. The patient had previously complained about treatment and this was possibly the reason for the defensive approach in the records.

In fact, though, this patient was seriously ill. There was a lack of proper information in the records. There was nothing recorded about the patient's history, planned treatment, planned care or procedures that had been carried out. Following a change of shift the new staff had no idea what was going on with the patient and this resulted in the patient's care being compromised.

The patient made a complaint. There was no useful information in the records and as a result the Trust could not defend the matter. The health professional who failed to make appropriate entries was called to account.

Writing records in this defensive way can be detrimental to the patient and makes the health professional who wrote them vulnerable to legal and professional consequences.

Records used in evidence are explored later in the book.

RECORD KEEPING IS A CHORE

Record keeping is often seen as a chore. Amongst the demands and pressures of a busy working day, it gets in the way of the hands-on tasks of direct contact with the patient. This view is clearly wrong and shows a lack of understanding of the nature of the health professionals' responsibility. If the health professional does not see it in this way it will be reflected in the records.

It is often said by health professionals, 'I am too busy to write the records'. You do not want to be the health professional standing in the witness box saying 'I'm sorry the patient died, but I didn't have time to write the records'!

More importantly, you do not want to be the health professional responsible for causing the death of the patient because you did not have the time the write the records.

> **SCENARIO**
>
> The patient is seen and assessed. The health professional decides on care and planned treatment and in the meantime the patient requires analgesia for pain relief.
>
> The health professional would never dream of dealing with a patient by taking a history, deciding on care and then saying, 'I will give you an analgesic, but I am a bit busy today. Maybe if I have time later or maybe tomorrow I will give you pain relief.'
>
> That would be preposterous and we would never treat the patient that way. Yet too often health professionals think that hands-on care is paramount and that record keeping does not form part of the care of the patient.

A health professional has an obligation to maintain the records. For example, the NMC guidelines state that 'record keeping is a tool of professional practice and one that should help the care process. It is not separate from this process and it is not an optional extra to be fitted in if circumstances allow.'[6]

The approach, 'I will complete the records later if I have time', which is often taken, is clearly wrong.

Consider the previous scenario. Writing the records is all part of the same process. It is as important as the hands-on care and should not be seen as separate from that. In the same way that the care and treatment of the patient is planned the health professional must also plan the documentation because the documents are part of the planned care. It is a tool of professional practice and one that should help the care process. It is not separate or distinct from the care process. They are both part of the same process.

In my experience as a trainer, the response by health professionals is that in theory they would like to write the records, but the demands of their role, lack of resources and lack of staff, etc., means that they simply cannot find the time. I sympathise with health professionals on this score, but nevertheless the health professional who says, 'I am too busy to write the records', will find themselves accountable. Being 'too busy' is not a defence. Remember, the court's view is that if it isn't recorded then it didn't happen, was not said or was not done.

In practice, health professionals need to look at their current regime for record keeping and time management to see where adjustments can be made to ease this process. Further guidance in this chapter will help health professionals to adjust and adapt their practices to the pressures they are now faced with so that they do not compromise their patients or themselves.

WHAT CONSTITUTES THE HEALTH RECORDS AND LEGAL DOCUMENTS?

What constitutes a health record and legal document? When does a health record become a legal document?

All documents relating to the health of a patient constitute a health record. They may include the following:

➤ clinical records
➤ nursing records
➤ nursing care plans
➤ therapy notes such as physiotherapy or occupational therapy

➤ assessments
➤ correspondence
➤ test results
➤ x-rays
➤ scans
➤ GP records
➤ community care records
➤ social work records
➤ counselling records.

In addition to the health records, other records may constitute a legal document and may be required to be produced before the court. These documents include:
➤ nursing kardex
➤ diaries
➤ handover notes
➤ theatre lists
➤ reports general or relating to a patient
➤ complaints file
➤ internal memorandum
➤ emails
➤ faxes.

In that past I have seen, in midwifery records, a paper hand towel or the nurse's apron with time of delivery written on it. The apron and hand towel form part of the record and should be retained, regardless of whether it has also been written in the records. However, writing on aprons and paper hand towels is not best practice.

Any document may be requested by the court. Therefore, anything you write in relation to patients' healthcare may be disclosed to the court. Any document relating to the case can be requested or subpoenaed by the court.

Records that are unconnected with the patient may be requested. For example, in the case of Deacon v McVicar 1984 QBD,[7] there was a dispute about the priority given to a patient. The court ordered that the records of other patients on the ward be disclosed so that it could assess whether or not other patients were making demands on medical and nursing staff at a particular time.

If the records or documentation cannot be found then the Trust will have to explain to the court the details of searches made and the circumstances of their disappearance.

WHO SHOULD WRITE THE RECORDS?

The health professional carrying out the care is responsible for writing the entry in the records. This extends to unregistered staff, such as healthcare assistants, who have first-hand knowledge of the patient's care.

Delegating the documentation of records

Although those who are providing the care are responsible for recording the entries in the records, sometimes the health professional will delegate the writing of entries in the records to another member of staff; for example, during the ward round the consultant may delegate the task of writing the entry in the records to the junior doctor.[8]

The danger of this is that the junior doctor will not have the same level of knowledge as the consultant and may misunderstand some of the detail, or treatment planned, etc. The responsibility for making sure that the information is correct falls on both the consultant and the junior doctor. The consultant should always check the entry in the record to ensure that the information is correct to avoid a breakdown of communication and so avoid compromising the patient's care. The junior doctor should clarify with the consultant any information about which they are unsure.

In some Trusts, the policy is that the consultant should write their own notes. This is best practice.

EXAMPLE OF THE DANGER OF DELEGATING THE WRITING OF RECORD ENTRIES

In one scenario, it came to the attention of the consultant that there was a problem with the ward round notes when all 15 patients on a ward had the same history, same diagnosis and the same planned care. It then became apparent that the junior doctor was unable to keep up with the consultant on the ward round and had made the same entry in each set of records.

Healthcare assistants are often prohibited from writing the care they deliver in the records, notwithstanding the fact that they provide much of the patient's care. It is the supervisor who then writes up the care provided by the healthcare assistant in the notes. Such an entry will look as if it is the supervisor who has actually delivered the care when, in fact, they have not.

Some Trusts do allow healthcare assistants to record their own notes. This avoids any potential error in the records. In these circumstances the health professional, or supervisor, could countersign the entry to show that the appropriate care has been provided according to the records.

WHEN SHOULD THE RECORDS BE WRITTEN?

TASK 5.2

- When do you write your notes?
- When do you think they should be written?

There are a variety of time lines when health professionals state that the records are actually made. They include:

1. at the end of the shift
2. within 24 hours
3. as soon as practicable
4. contemporaneously
5. when returning from coffee break
6. at the end of the morning and again in the afternoon
7. when they get a break
8. whilst with the patient in his home
9. in the car between visits to patients
10. back at the office
11. on Monday after the weekend
12. not at all, when the patient has specifically requested that the information should not be disclosed because the information is confidential or the patient has asked you not write it down.

By far the easiest and safest way to record is by writing up the records contemporaneously; that is, 'at the same time'. The health professional making the record at the end of the shift or at the end of the day may spend an hour or two on this task. This then becomes a chore and they are less likely to record the detail – and may even confuse one patient's notes with another. Therefore the delay in documenting could compromise the patient's care.

By spending a few extra moments with the patient to make the entries, the health professional saves the two hours or so added to the end of their day. The entry is likely to reflect more accurately the detail and as there is no delay there is less likely to be a breakdown of communication.

However, there are occasions when it is not always possible or appropriate to write 'at the same time'; for example, in mental health where the health professional is conducting a 'listening session'. It is part of the treatment to 'listen to the patient', thus to write at the same time when listening to the patient may hinder the patient's treatment.

In obstetric care it would not be practical to ask the mother to stop pushing, seconds before delivery, so that the health professional can make a record! Although in some obstetric units they do have a designated note taker who records the whole process to ensure accurate and contemporaneous records. I suspect this is not common practice in the majority of maternity units due to cost and lack of resources.

The main reason for writing contemporaneously is to ensure the patient's care is not compromised. The longer the delay before writing the records, the more likely it is that the health professional will forget the detail. There is a danger that the entries will then become routine and meaningless and it is more likely that there will be a breakdown in communication. The health professional will be dealing with similar patients with similar conditions, which makes it easier to make a mistake between one patient's notes and another's. Their individual details may erroneously merge, or the details may simply have been forgotten by the time it is recorded.

There is an inherent danger in letting time elapse between contact with the patient and making an entry, as the following examples show.

EXAMPLES OF THE CONSEQUENCES OF DELAYED RECORDING KEEPING

1   What would happen if you attend to a patient, but decide to have your coffee break before making the entry in the record?

    The patient is then seen by another health professional who is now ignorant of the information you have in your head. This may result in the other health professional treating the patient inappropriately. The patient's care may be compromised.

2 What about the health visitor whose practice it is to see patients Monday to Friday, but not write up the records for the week until Friday afternoon? What happens if she is hit by a bus on Thursday night?
There are no records for the week!

We can see from these examples the inherent dangers of delaying making entries in records. Remember, the longer it is left the more likely it is that the detail will be missed and the higher the risk of a breakdown of communication.

HOW MUCH SHOULD BE WRITTEN?

How much should be written in the records is determined by the quality of the information and not the quantity of the entries. There is little point in writing for the sake of it if the records do not tell us anything.

EXAMPLE OF UNNECESSARY INFORMATION

A patient had been admitted for a surgical procedure requiring an over-night admission. The entries in the record consisted of nursing records of around seven pages. The records read along the lines of:

'I saw the patient and she told me she wants a bar of chocolate. The patient then went to get a bar a chocolate and the patient gave me a dirty look on the stairs witnessed by Sandra.'

'Patient wants to go outside and have a fag' and 'patient wants to telephone her mother . . .'

How useful was this information? What does it tell us about the patient's condition, planned care or treatment? Well, in fact, nothing at all.

There was no information about planned care, the operation or the patient's condition. How frustrating is it for the health professional to have to read seven pages of these types of notes and discover at the end that there is no useful information contained within the record? The health professional is already under time pressure and this is a waste of time for both the writer and the reader.

Deciding on how much to write will largely depend on professional judgment in your field of expertise. The health professional will know the kind of information, the signs and symptoms that they are looking for, what history to extract and so on. A useful yardstick to use when deciding how much to write is to ask yourself this question: 'If I was going to a patient for the first time, what would I need to know?' This will enable you to judge the relevance of the entries.

Remember, your records will be shared with other health professionals. If, for some reason, you are prevented from returning to work through sickness, holiday or maternity leave, for example, it should make no difference to the care the patient will receive. Someone reading your notes should be able to pick up from where you left off. The next health professional may be a student, agency staff, locum or new member of staff. They need to be able to easily pick up the information in the records and continue with patient care.

WHAT SHOULD BE WRITTEN?

The NMC guidelines on record keeping state that the best record is one that is the product of the consultation and discussion that has taken place at a local level between all members of the inter-professional healthcare team and the patient.

The best record is one that enables a health professional to care for the patient, regardless of where they are within the care process or care environment. It is an invaluable way of promoting communication within the healthcare team and between practitioners and their patients. Therefore, good record keeping is both the product of good teamwork and an important tool for promoting high quality healthcare. Patients should be equal partners, whenever possible, in the compilation of their own records.

There is no national agreement between all healthcare professions on standards and format of records. There is no rigid framework, no one way of recording information, so I cannot set out a black-and-white system for recording health records. The records may differ depending on the needs of the patient. One might imagine that it would be common sense for the format and content for all healthcare records to be the same across all healthcare providers. This would greatly assist in the event that a patient moves to a new geographical area. Thus the new health providers would be familiar with the documentation, which would make the transition of patient care easier and less likely to result in a breakdown of communication. This would also assist greatly with the movement of staff, whereby all staff would be familiar with the documentation if they moved to another Trust – thus removing confusion and the risk of breakdown in communication. However, in practice, this consistency of documentation does not exist. Community care documentation differs from acute care and even within them documentation varies between departments.

There have been attempts in the past to have a uniform national standard for documentation but it is very difficult to apply the motto 'one size fits all'. Computerisation may assist in standardising the documentation. Electronic records are discussed later in Chapter 14.

In the meantime, and in the absence of a rigid framework, this book will explore best practice. Remember, too, that there may be polices and guidelines set down at local level and by professional bodies and they should be read alongside the information set out in this chapter.

Whilst I cannot tell you in every circumstance what to write, I can tell you what to avoid, what should be included and what can be left out.

As with the length of the entry, deciding what to write and what is relevant will again largely come down to your professional judgment, your areas of expertise and knowledge. You will know the kinds of questions to ask to extract the history and information and the signs and symptoms that you are looking for.

As previously stated, the approach to record keeping that courts of law adopt is that 'if it is not recorded, then it has not been done or was not said'. This applies particularly to situations where the condition of the patient is apparently unchanging and no record has been made of the care delivered. Local standards should be set down to define how frequently the notes should record that there has been no change.

Patient records should be clear, accurate, unambiguous, factual and consistent. They should be written in terms that the patient can understand.

WHAT TO INCLUDE

The records should give an account of:
➤ current information on the care and condition of the patient
➤ what the health professional tells the patient
➤ the treatment given
➤ the effectiveness of the treatment

➤ the problems that have arisen and the action taken to rectify
  them
➤ the care planned, the decisions made, the care delivered and the
  information shared
➤ the actions agreed with the patient (including consent to treatment
  and/or consent to share the records)
➤ observations (examinations, tests, diagnoses, prognoses, prescriptions,
  other treatments) including negative findings
➤ disclosures by the patient relevant to understanding cause or effect of
  cure/treatment
➤ facts presented to the patient, including information and health
  promotion leaflets
➤ correspondence from the patient or other parties
➤ information about hyper-sensitivity (allergic) reactions and other
  information written in a designated part of the record and relevant to
  all healthcare professionals
➤ times, dates, authentication (i.e. signature, name printed in full and
  designation).

WHAT TO OMIT

The records should not include:

➤ jargon
➤ meaningless phrases
➤ irrelevant speculation
➤ offensive and subjective statements
➤ personal opinions regarding the patient, which should be restricted to
  professional judgments on clinical matters
➤ complaints from the patient, which should be held in a separate file.

DON'T KEEP IT IN YOUR HEAD

'You are not looking yourself today; that wound is not getting any better.'

Don't make a mental record. A mental record fades quickly in its accuracy
and this is why we use written records. Remember – written records are communication tools. There is a real danger that when we become familiar with

the patient we do not record the level of detail that we should. We may know the patient well and may have seen the patient daily. We may, for example, look at the patient's wound and know that it is better than it was yesterday. The danger is that because we are familiar with the patient we fail to record the detail. The records then lack the detail necessary for other health professionals to continue with patient care.

EXAMPLES OF KEEPING ONLY A MENTAL RECORD

The health professional may attend the patient daily and clean and dress the wound. That health professional is familiar with how the wound is progressing and enters a record that reads, 'wound dressed'. But how will the next health professional know if the wound is getting better or worse or if the current treatment is working when there is nothing in the notes to measure it by?

Another example is illustrated in the case study in Chapter 4, when the consultant made a diagnosis but 'kept it in the back of his mind' and did not record it in the notes. This had serious consequences for patient care.

The records are a tool for communicating. The health professional will be relying upon them. How will your colleagues know what is going on with the patient if you keep the information in your head? This compromises patient care and you will be accountable. So don't keep it in your head – record it!

HEALTH RECORDS SHOULD INCLUDE . . .

The records should be written in terms the patient can understand and should be written wherever possible with the involvement of the patient.

Health professionals should consider including the following information in the records:

➤ **GP's details** – including name, address, telephone number and GP identification number.
➤ **Admission details** – date and time of admission, route of admission, type of admission (e.g. emergency or elective), source of admission and name of referring GP.
➤ **Reason for admission** – (e.g. clinical review, referral by GP).
➤ **Presenting problem** – signs, symptoms, condition, or if this is not applicable, the reason for admission should be recorded.

➤ **History of presenting problem** – how long the patient has had the symptoms or the condition.

➤ **Current diagnosis** – disorders, syndromes, diseases the patient currently suffers from.

➤ **Allergies** – allergies the person suffers from, including hyper-sensitivities. There should be a designated place in the records for recording allergies.

➤ **Past illnesses** – including previous disorders, syndromes and diseases that do not currently affect the patient. Dates should be included.

➤ **Procedures and investigations** – any operations or investigations the patient has had.

➤ **Medications and diets** – any substance the patient is taking regularly or as required; consider also herbal remedies. Include the dose, frequency and route of administration and duration for each medication.

➤ **Social circumstances** – domestic and employment lifestyle information.

➤ **Family history** – any relevant family history.

➤ **Examination finding** – include general observations, pulse rate, blood pressure and temperature, as well as assessment of cardiovascular, respiratory or nervous systems.

➤ **Results of investigations** – test results, assessments, identification of problems and action to be taken. Differential diagnoses should be recorded with planned care until the diagnosis is made.

➤ **Overall assessments** – clinicians' overall assessment of the patient's condition. If there is 'no change' then this may be recorded.

➤ **Problem lists** – identify the patient's problems.

➤ **Management plans** – procedures or medication to resolve the problems identified. Include plans for review and follow up. When following up, if the plan has not changed since the last entry then 'continue' can be recorded. Any changes in the plan and new problems must be recorded.

➤ **Care planned** – care planned, decisions made, care delivered and information shared. Identify problems that have arisen and action taken to rectify them.

➤ **Source of information** – (e.g. from examination) the patient, relative, translator or ambulance service.

➤ **Intended outcomes** – include prognosis.

➤ **Treatment given** – including the type and dosage of drugs, total amount prescribed and any other treatment.

➤ **Information given to the patient** – any information given to the patient or their families about their condition, care, etc.

➤ **Follow-up entries** – every follow-up entry should record clearly what has happened or been done to the patient since the previous entry, the assessment of the patient's condition, new management plan and information given to the patient.

➤ **Reason for clinical encounter** – this may include, for example, 'ward round' or 'asked to see the patient'.

➤ **Review of case** – this should include any new information that relates to the patient.

➤ **People present** – nurse, chaperone, interpreter, team in a multi-disciplinary meeting or family member.

➤ **Comments and statements** – all comments, statements, questions and answers by the patient (particularly when dealing with consent issues).

➤ **Advanced directives** – these must be clearly recorded in the notes alongside any resuscitation statements.

➤ **Discharge/transfer** – when a patient is transferred or discharged there must be communication with those involved in the patient's care. The patient must be informed as to what information will be communicated and their consent for disclosure must be obtained. Copies of any communication should be retained in the records. *See* Chapter 13 under the section 'Copying letters to GPs and patients'. Discharge or transfer summaries should contain details of the patient's GP, admission details, review of the case, current diagnosis, allergies, procedures and investigations, medications and diet, examination findings, results of investigations, problem lists, management plan, intended outcomes and information given to the patient. Discharge summaries should be validated by a senior clinician. Discharge summaries should be multidisciplinary where multidisciplinary care is to be continued.

REFERENCES

1 The Nursing and Midwifery Council. *Midwives' Rules and Standards*. Available at: www.nmc-uk.org/aFrameDisplay.aspx?DocumentID=169 (accessed 10 February 2009).
2 www.mhac.org.uk
3 www.mwcscot.org.uk
4 www.mhcni.org
5 Royal College of Nursing. Good record keeping is vital. *East Midlands News*. 13 September 2006.

6 The Nursing and Midwifery Council. *Guidelines for Records and Record Keeping*; 2005. Available at: www.nmc-uk.org/aFrameDisplay.aspx?DocumentID=4008 (accessed 10 February 2009).

7 Deacon v McVicar 1984 unreported QBD.

8 General Medical Council. *Good Medical Practice*; 2006. Available at: www.gmc-uk.org/guidance/good_medical_practice/index.asp (accessed 11 February 2009).

CHAPTER 6

The detail

Health records should be clear, factual, consistent and accurate. It is the detail that is important as it tells us about what is going on with the patient. If we do not note down the details then the records will be meaningless. The difficulty is knowing just how much detail to note down.

It is often the lack of detail that causes a problem with records. If we do not write the details there is a danger we will miss something; for example, the subtle changes in a patient's condition.

Words can have a huge impact. If you fail to record with clarity then the patient's care may be compromised. It is important to think about what is being written. When you write the records, reflect on them and think about whether others will know what you mean. Are your records clear?

INADEQUATE DETAIL

Where there is a failure to record adequate detail the communication between health professionals will be hampered. Undue reliance may be placed on limited detail and an appropriate diagnosis can easily be missed. Whether to record the minutiae of detail depends on whether it is deemed important by the health professional. The health professional might record a verbatim account where seemingly small details assume greater significance; for example, where risk to the patient is an issue, self-harm, child abuse or abuse of a vulnerable adult.

THE RATIONALE

A common error in the records is to omit the rationale (i.e. the reason for the treatment). Health professionals go through the correct process and reach a professional judgment based on the clinical picture and other details, but then only record the outcome and fail to record the rationale for how they got to that point.

The difficulty is that when we make a decision about patient care but fail to record the rationale, the next health professional caring for the patient will not have the full picture and so may not make the correct decision.

EXAMPLE OF THE ABSENCE OF THE RATIONALE

The health professional takes the history from the patient, examines the patient and then decides on planned care. The health professional decides that the patient should be administered antibiotic.

If the entry in the health records simply reads 'commenced antibiotic' without the rationale, the next health professional who cares for the patient will be in the dark. They will not know why the patient has been administered antibiotic, how much antibiotic has been administered, when the antibiotic started and how long it is to continue.

In the absence of the rationale recorded in the notes it is difficult for any health professional to decide on the patient's future care.

In the above example, because the subsequent health professional has no idea why antibiotics were administered in the first instance, they may make a decision to withdraw the antibiotics. This health professional will not be able to make a judgment as to any change of dose that might be appropriate.

In reality, the health professional may go through the correct process but not record it. The health professional takes a history from the patient, examines the patient and decides on a course of treatment or planned care. However, what sometimes happens is that the health professional records only the outcome. Remember, the health professional is accountable for the entry in the record. If the writer were to visit the documentation sometime after patient care has been provided, that health professional will have difficulty in recalling why they acted in a particular way.

CLARITY OF DETAIL

Often recorded in the notes are vague words or phrases like 'normal' or 'appears ok' and 'not too bad'. How will other health professionals understand what is meant? What does 'normal' mean? The word 'appears' could have several meanings and each health professional may place their own interpretation on it. Entries should be clear and factual.

EXAMPLE OF VAGUE REFERENCES

The patient presents with pain in her left wrist following a fall. She is examined, an x-ray is taken and the results show that there is no fracture or break. The entry in the record should reflect this. If the only words entered were 'appears OK', the next health professional would have no idea what they mean, what tests were carried out and what the results of those tests were.

The health professional needs to consider what led them to believe that the patient's condition was 'normal' or 'appears ok'. Then we need to go back and consider what the facts were that led us to believe that it was 'normal' or 'appears ok'. It is the factual information – the rationale – that we need to record and not simply the outcome or the decision.

Lack of clarity in the detail of the meaning of words compromises patient care. It exposes the health professionals – both the reader and the writer – to problems with legal and professional accountability.

EXAMPLE OF TWO TYPES OF RECORDS

Consider the following two sets of records. The patient's blood pressure and temperature are taken. During a period of an hour and a half there are changes in the blood pressure and temperature, but they are within the normal range.

Have a look at Record No 1. If you were presented with this entry would you have concerns? Would you feel it necessary to react?

Record No 1

Date	Clinical notes (*each entry must be signed*)
27/08/06	
12.00	Normal

| 12.30 | Normal |
| 13.00 | Normal |

On the face of this record there is nothing that would concern the health professional and further action is unlikely to be implemented.

Would your reaction alter if the entry were presented differently?

Have a look at Record no 2. If you were presented with this entry would you
have concerns? Would you feel it necessary to react?

Record No 2

Date	Clinical notes (*each entry must be signed*)
27/08/06	
12.00	BP 140/90 t 37
12.30	BP 130/85 t 37.5
13.00	BP 120/80 t 38

In Record no 2 the detail of the blood pressure and temperature is recorded. We
can see from this entry that although the blood pressure and temperature are
within the normal range, the blood pressure is dropping and the temperature
is increasing. We can see that these changes have occurred over a period of
an hour and a half. It is more likely that the health professional will question the
condition of the patient based on this record. Is this the onset of an infection?
Does another health professional need to be involved? Do antibiotics need to
be administered?

From this illustration we can see the impact of the way in which the information is presented. The lack of detail in Record No 1 may result in a failure to
treat the patient appropriately. It takes little extra effort to write the details
than to write the word 'normal'.

EXAMPLE OF AN INADEQUATE RECORD

Lack of detail is a significant problem. Consider a typical entry in the record that
reads 'wound cleaned and dressed'.

The patient is seen by various district nurses every day for five days. The
entries read as follows:

Date	Clinical notes (*each entry must be signed*)
01/09/06	Wound cleaned and dressed
11.00	J. Smith
02/09/06	Wound cleaned and dressed
11.00	J. Smith
03/09/06	Wound cleaned and dressed
11.00	T. Turner
04/09/06	Wound cleaned and dressed
11.00	M. Loe
05/09/06	Wound cleaned and dressed
11.00	B. Jones
06/09/06	Wound infected requires admission ambulance called
11.00	J. Smith

This entry shows that several health professionals attended the patient daily to clean the wound and to change the patient's dressing. How then did this patient develop an infection resulting in hospital admission?

The reason is simply that there is no useful description of the wound. How do the district nurses know whether the wound is getting better or worse if there is nothing to measure it by?

The purpose of the record is not simply to show that the district nurses visited each day. The records are there for the benefit of the patient, for their care and treatment. An entry like 'wound sloughy in the centre for one centimetre and red on the edges' would have enabled each health professional to measure the wound's progress.

Sadly, lack of detail in records is a common problem and one that could be avoided with good documentation. Consider the consequences of the example above. The patient is suffering, there is a delay in recovery – or worse, there could be serious or life-threatening consequences. Consider also the cost entailed in the transfer to hospital, admission and treatment, the potential claim for compensation the patient would have and the professional consequences for the health professionals involved.

CLEAR AND UNAMBIGUOUS

It is important that entries in the record are clear and unambiguous. Previously I mentioned that it is the quality of the information that is important rather than the quantity and that there is little point recording entries like 'patient wants to telephone her mother' or 'patient wants a bar of chocolate' when it does little to assist in patient care, planning or treatment. Of course some of those comments may, in some circumstances, be relevant. For example, if the patient had been advised to stay in bed but was insistent upon moving around against medical advice, this could impact on the patient's condition. If that is the case the records need to explain the relevance of such entries with detail of the risks and advice given.

The rest of this chapter covers what should be recorded when considering the detail.

CARE AND CONDITION

The records should demonstrate the care and the condition of the patient, the treatment that has been given and the effectiveness of the treatment, and should provide evidence of the care planned. This needs to include the decisions made, the care delivered and the information shared with others. The records must provide evidence of actions agreed with the patient, including consent to treatment and/or consent to share the records.

Failure to document care given is often a source of complaint by a patient. The HSC Annual Report of 2003[1] reported a complaint regarding a failure to treat a myeloma patient adequately. They found that there was no evidence to suggest that appropriate nursing care planning or careful monitoring of the patient took place. The report stated that 'there were no written care plans or protocols to provide information for any of the staff about the management of the patient's condition'.

Current information on the care and condition of the patient should be recorded. This can be cross-referenced with other documents, such as charts. Whilst it is acceptable to cross-reference with other documentation, remember your record is a tool for communicating. If there is something that is important, simply cross-referencing the documentation may result in the health professional missing something. For example, the patient may have increasing temperature and decreasing blood pressure. Because the health professional is concerned about this, it would be prudent to make an entry in the clinical record to highlight this rather than simply stating in the record 'see chart'. It is important to alert other health professionals to any concerns.

ADVICE GIVEN

You should document the detail of what you tell the patient and the advice you give to the patient.

This should include:

➤ the facts presented to the patient
➤ the detail of the advice given
➤ details of any leaflets given to the patient (include the name of the leaflets)
➤ any emphasis on advice (e.g. the patient may have an underlying condition of diabetes, so in addition to the usual advice, further advice may have been given because of this condition. It is important to document this)
➤ if the patient does not want to accept the advice then that should be recorded and if possible the reasons why be given.

CASE STUDY

In one case, the HSC[1] investigated a complaint about a woman who had died without being told that she was seriously ill with cancer. An entry in the records said that Mrs L had been told about the possibility of cancer and other staff said they had discussed Mrs L's condition with Mr L. However, they had not recorded these conversations. It was therefore not clear what information had been given to Mr L or what language was used to convey it. One of the HSC recommendations was that conversations with patients and relatives should be documented.

ADVICE AND CONSENT

As part of patient care, health professionals will give advice to patients and part of that advice is informing the patient of the risks involved in the various treatment options. It is not sufficient simply to record in the notes 'patient advised of risks'. This does not provide enough information for other health professionals dealing with the care of the patient to ascertain precisely what was discussed. Details of the risks you advised the patient of must be recorded. For example, the patient may have been informed of the known risks of a particular procedure, but may not have been informed of the risks due to a pre-existing underlying condition, such as diabetes or a heart problem. If the entry in the record simply reads 'patient advised of risks', then the health professionals involved in the patient care and treatment may make an assumption that the patient had been advised of all of those risks, when in fact the patient had not.

This has significant implications for issues of consent, which may render consent invalid. More importantly, the purpose of documenting the risks is to ensure that the patient has been fully advised so that they can then make a decision regarding their care.

When a problem arises relating to consent, if there is a dispute as to what risks were discussed, the records will be relied on in order to resolve the dispute. If the record only states 'patient advised of risks', the patient later may say, for example, 'you told me that I might get an infection, but you did not tell me that I might bleed, and had I known that I would not have had the procedure'. This highlights one of the problems that can be faced by health professionals in failing to document fully.

The consent forms may consist of tick boxes. A tick box may read 'has the patient been advised of the risks?' This tick box lacks the detail required. It is now more common in standard forms to see the words, 'I confirm the patient has been advised of the following risks . . .' The detailed advice given in respect of the risks is then clearly recorded.

It is not a defence to say, 'The reason I did not record the detail was that there was no room on the form'. If there is no room on the form you should write the detail of your advice in the records.

When giving the patient advice you should also include in the records the advice given in relation to the consequences of not having treatment and the risks of this.

Advice might consist of leaflets. The content of the leaflet may have been explained to the patient and the patient may have been given leaflets to take away with them. This should be recorded in the notes along with the title of the leaflet, so that it is clear what advice has been given.

ACTION

A common error in the records is where the health professional identifies a problem but fails to detail any action to rectify this. Entries like 'chase test results' – but nobody obtains the results. The records are silent on who will actually chase for those results. There is an assumption that someone else is dealing with this or someone else will follow it up.

It is important that once a problem has been identified the detail of the action is clearly set out in the records. In addition it should identify who will follow through the action.

Often the records identify the problem such as 'suffering increased pain' or 'finding it difficult to swallow' and whilst action may actually have been taken there is often a failure to record it.

NEGATIVE FINDINGS

Records should include both positive and negative findings. Health professionals should take care not to exclude negative findings. They should, for example, record concerns raised by a patient's relatives. Relatives are often well placed to observe departures from a patient's usual pattern of behaviour, yet their comments are not always taken seriously or even recorded.

CASE STUDY

In the case of Johnston v Southport & Ormskirk Hospital NHS Trust,[2] it was alleged by the claimant that the hospital had been negligent by failing to diagnose breast cancer in 1999.

The court criticised the record keeping of one of the hospital doctors who saw Mrs Johnston, as inadequate. Mrs Johnston had raised concerns regarding her symptoms. The doctor had ruled out the concerns she raised but did not record this in the records. It should not be forgotten that one of the purposes of clinical notes is to assist others who may see the patient at a later date. To record that a patient's specific concern has been excluded would be of enormous assistance.

Health professionals would be well advised to study the above case and put into effect the judge's pertinent comments on the recording of negative findings in the notes where a patient has raised specific concerns.

FREQUENCY OF THE ENTRIES

The NMC guidelines[3] on record keeping state that the frequency of entries will be determined both by the professional judgment of the health professional and local standards and agreements. Health professionals will need to exercise particular care and make more frequent entries when patients present with complex problems, show deviation from the norm, require more intensive care than normal, are confused and disorientated or generally give cause for concern. They must use their professional judgment (if necessary in discussion with other members of the healthcare team) to determine when these circumstances exist.

SPELLING AND GRAMMAR

Health professionals must ensure that their spelling and grammar are accurate. Spelling and grammatical errors can result in a breakdown in communication and lead to mistakes in patient care. Decimal points in the wrong place have also led to errors in patient care. It was reported that a baby died as a result of a drug dose error due to the decimal point being in the wrong place in the records.[4]

In December 2001, it was reported in *The Times* that a typing error by a secretary is believed to have led to a transplant patient being given an incompatible kidney. The kidney had been donated by one of the patient's relatives, but was found not to be a match. A secretary is thought to have keyed the wrong laboratory matching-test results into a computer and the transplant went ahead. As a consequence the patient's body rejected the organ. The patient is now on dialysis and it is thought that it may be more difficult to match her for a transplant in the future.[5]

Even in computerised systems spelling errors can prove fatal. For example, it was reported that a spelling error might have cost a student her life. The omission of the letter 'P' in the surname of Charlotte Simpkin led to a doctor failing to obtain the pathology results of the patient. She had been admitted to hospital with suspected meningitis. She was given an injection of antibiotics by the GP, but the antibiotics were withdrawn shortly after admission to hospital when blood tests showed no sign of meningitis and a new diagnosis was made of a viral infection. An inquiry revealed that the results had been entered onto the computer under the wrong spelling of the patient's surname and were therefore not seen by the doctor. Criticisms were also made of communications systems between the pathology and medical staff.[6]

MISSING INFORMATION

If the health professional fails to record important information this can also lead to patient care being compromised. It could have detrimental consequences for the patient and professional repercussions for the health professional. For example, if the health professional were to leave out of the record the administration of a drug, this could mislead other health professionals and as a consequence the patient could be given an overdose.

Accurate, comprehensive information relating to the care and condition of the patient is a vital part of the role of the health professional. In addition, the information could be used for many other purposes of which the health professional may not be aware at the time.

Remember, the court's view is that 'if it is not recorded then it didn't happen, wasn't said or wasn't done'.

PATIENT'S DETAILS

It is important to record the patient's details on each page. You may think this is obvious, but it is surprising how many times this information is either not recorded or it is inaccurately recorded.

Patient information should include the following:
➤ the patient's full name
➤ the patient's date of birth
➤ the patient's identification number.
This information should be recorded on every page.

REFERENCES

1 Department of Health, Health Service Commissioner. *Annual Report 2003–4* E.2193/01–2.
2 Johnston v Southport & Ormskirk Hospital NHS Trust, Manchester County Court, 11/5/04. Available at: www.cr.rsmjournals.com/cgi/reprint/11/2/89-a.pdf
3 The Nursing and Midwifery Council. *Guidelines for Records and Record Keeping;* 2005.

Available at: www.nmc-uk.org/aFrameDisplay.aspx?DocumentID=4008 (accessed 10 February 2009).

4 Hurst G. Baby dies after one decimal point drug dose error. *The Times*. 11 October 2000.

5 Harris G. Patient given wrong kidney in typing error. *The Times*. 4 December 2001.

6 Johnstone H. Spelling mistake may have cost student her life. *The Times*. 28 August 1998.

CHAPTER 7

How do we record?

PROTOCOLS AND GUIDELINES

If when caring for a patient you are following protocols or guidelines, then you should record this in the records. This is particularly important in light of the issues surrounding, for example, infection control. If possible, a copy of the policy, protocol or guidelines referred to should remain with the records (depending on its volume). You should at least cross-reference your records with the policy, protocol or guidelines. Your records should demonstrate that the policy, protocol or guidelines are, in fact, being adhered to.

Where the policy or guidelines are not contained within the patient record then the health professional must know where they are kept.

Policies and guidelines are updated from time to time. It is important that you are able to demonstrate that you were following the policy or guidelines that were in place at that particular time.

If there is any departure from the protocol or guidelines when treating the patient, this must be clearly documented. You should state where you have departed from the protocol or guidelines, in what way and the rationale behind such a decision. You will be accountable for such decisions and you will therefore need to substantiate them.

The court will wish to see a copy of the policy, protocol or guidelines.

AGGRESSION

I often see entries in the record that state the patient was 'aggressive'. Aggression can manifest itself in many ways. For example, the pointing of a finger can feel very intimidating and aggressive. Alternatively, the patient may be aggressive and demonstrates this by waving a machete. Pointing a finger and waving a machete are two ends of the scale so the word 'aggressive' does not really demonstrate what is meant. Therefore, it is appropriate to write in the record how this aggression is manifesting itself. A more detailed description will be required. You may state in the records: 'The patient was aggressive; for example, the patient asked me for a glass of water and at the same time threw a glass at me, which hit the wall behind me and shattered into pieces'.

It is important to document such detail in order to assess risk for the protection of the patient and others. For example, in community care, because of the aggression the decision may be made that health professionals should be accompanied when attending the patient's home. In the absence of detail in the documentation of the aggression, such decisions will be difficult to make and justify and could place others at risk.

FAILURE BY THE PATIENT TO COMPLY

When the patient does not wish to accept advice of the health professionals, refuses to take medication or acts in a particular way that is contrary to medical advice, it is particularly important to set this out in detail. The record should clearly state the advice given, the way in which the patient is non-compliant, why the patient is non-compliant if that information is available, details of the risks of such non-compliance and whether the patient has been informed of those risks.

THIRD PARTY INFORMATION

Health professionals are sometimes reticent about writing information when it has come from someone other than the patient themselves.

The health professional should record the facts. If they have received information, the notes should record the information given and the name of the person who gave it. If a family member tells the health professional something about a patient, it should state in the records who told them. The health professional should not exclude the person's name for fear of breaching confidentiality. There are measures in place to deal with issues of confidentiality should they arise.

If the information from a third person places the patient at risk, the information should not be excluded, but can be dealt with by way of a supplementary record. For example, where a family member tells you something, but if you were to record the name of the family member and what they said in the patient-held record, this may result in the health professional being refused entry into the home. This could place the patient at risk. An example of this is where a patient is terminally ill and is being cared for at home by her son and being visited by health visitors. The patient tells the health visitor that her son is a known drug user and is taking her morphine. To put this information in the patient-held record would alert the son who may then refuse the health visitor entry.

TELEPHONE ADVICE

Health professionals are often in the position of giving or receiving information and advice over the telephone, either with other health professionals or patients.

How should this be recorded and who should record it?

Increasingly, health professionals are giving advice over the telephone. GPs, doctors, infection-control nurses or supervisors, for example, may receive a telephone call from another health professional for advice on how to treat or care for a patient. In these circumstances the advisor may not have the records to hand and so will not be in a position to make a contemporaneous note in the records. The advisor should ask the health professional seeking the advice to make a note in the records. The advisor should ask the health professional to read back to them the entry that they have made. This is not to cover the backs of the advisors or health professionals, but rather to ensure that the advisor has understood the presenting details and the health professional has understood the advice. This will avoid any misunderstandings and will ensure that the patient will receive the correct treatment. When asking the health professional to read back the entry they have made, it is surprising how many times you may hear or have to say, 'that is not what I meant' or 'that is not what I said'.

Included in the note should be details of what the health professional seeking advice has told the advisor about the patient. This will ensure the advisor asks the correct questions and gives appropriate advice. It is important that signs and symptoms are clearly described to compensate for not having a face-to-face meeting with the patient.

A health professional may give telephone advice directly to the patient. A contemporaneous note should be made directly into the records. If the records are not to hand, the details should be recorded ideally on a telephone advice note and this should then be physically placed into the records themselves. Alternatively, a note may be made as an aide-memoire and the information should then be written into the records as soon as possible.

When obtaining the details from the patient, think carefully about how the patient describes their symptoms. You should explore the detail to ensure that you have asked the necessary questions and obtained all the necessary details in order to give appropriate advice.

When advising a patient the record should include the following:
➤ the patient's name
➤ date of birth
➤ hospital number or address
➤ telephone number
➤ usual partner or carer
➤ permission to discuss information with partner or carer should there be a need to return the call
➤ current problem
➤ specific advice
➤ details of diagnosis, current treatment, monitoring, medical inventions and dates of any future appointments
➤ all medicines, including over the counter and complementary therapies
➤ any relevant social or psychological issues
➤ what was agreed, including time frame, advice given if problem continues and any steps for follow-up.

The following case illustrates the hazards of diagnosing over the telephone.

CASE STUDY

Oliver was born prematurely and developed hydrocephalus, which is an abnormal amount of cerebrospinal fluid around the brain. A tube was fitted to drain the excess fluid from his skull, in order to avoid excessive pressure building up within the brain. Oliver's condition was well documented within his GP records and he had experienced difficulties with the tube blocking on previous occasions, which had been acted upon quickly and treated.

Oliver complained of a headache and had vomited suddenly at school. His mother called their GP for advice and during a short telephone call the GP diagnosed a viral infection.

The following day Oliver's symptoms deteriorated and he was rushed to hospital where it was found that the tube in his skull was blocked. He suffered a cardiac arrest and the increased pressure in his skull had caused damage to his brain.

Oliver's mother and the GP's recollection of their telephone conversation were quite different. This discussion was considered in some detail during the court trial, which addressed whether the GP had provided Oliver with a reasonable level of care. Many issues arose including how Oliver's mother actually described his symptoms. Should the GP have asked specific questions to rule out a tube block? Was a visit to the GP and/or a home visit mandatory and did the GP take a satisfactory medical history?

The judge in this case found that the GP was in breach of his duty of care to Oliver by failing to take a sufficient history to exclude the possibility of a blocked tube. It would have been common sense for the GP to ask specific questions to exclude a tube blockage and there was no logical basis not to ask these. If this had been done, Oliver would have been referred to hospital a day earlier and his brain damage would have been prevented.

This judgment was given despite evidence from two GP experts that it was not negligent to fail to ask direct questions. Despite this, the judge substituted his own opinion that such an approach was not logical given Oliver's unique previous medical history and the problems with the tube.[1]

COMPLAINT

A complaint reported by the HSC identified that there was a failure to record a telephone call about a risk of suicide.

A father complained to the HSC[2] following the death by suicide of his daughter. She had a history of mental illness and had been detained under the Mental Health Act. She was given temporary home leave and the following day she took her own life.

The father was concerned that she had been given leave even though his partner had telephoned the centre the day before to express the fear that his daughter had been threatening to commit suicide. The call was neither recorded nor acted upon.

The HSC assessors concluded that the care plans were inadequate, that his daughter should have been nursed in a different environment and that the standard of documentation was poor. They also believed that the decision to grant leave was inappropriate.

The Trust agreed to review its nurse training programmes, to remind staff of the importance of recording and reporting significant external information, to issue new guidelines for record keeping and to remind staff of the need to involve relatives in patients' care.

This case illustrates the need to carefully record telephone calls and the dangers of poor record keeping.

A legal case may stand or fall on the basis of a simple telephone call.

SCENARIO

A patient had a history of back pain following injury in a road traffic accident. She also had a history of urinary problems. She suffered loss of bladder and bowel control on Friday afternoon. She telephoned the GP that afternoon. The GP advised, 'See how you get on over the weekend. If you are no better by Monday call the surgery'.

By Monday the patient's symptoms were no better. The GP was unable to give her an appointment on Monday morning so she took herself to A&E. A diagnosis of cauda equina syndrome was made. (The 'cauda equina' are the nerves at the base of the spine. Damage to them can result in loss of power and sensation in the legs and loss of bladder and bowel control. If not treated urgently, any such loss can be permanent.)

The patient underwent emergency surgery. However, the surgery was too late and the patient's loss of bowel and bladder control was permanent as a result of the delay.

There was nothing recorded in the GP notes about the telephone call made on Friday. The GP could not recall any such conversation taking place. However, the patient produced the telephone bill clearly showing that she had telephoned the surgery, with the call lasting around 15 minutes. It is likely that court will accept the patient's version of events. This is discussed in the later chapter notes as evidence.

Care needs to be taken when giving and receiving telephone advice and recording it.

The Royal College of Nursing has published guidance on telephone advice lines for people with long-term conditions,[3] which health professionals may find useful.

RECORDING CONSENT ISSUES

Consent is a complex topic and health professionals need to understand consent issues in order to document them appropriately. Not all consent issues will be written as some of them may be implied. Some consent issues may be recorded on standard forms and others written in the health records.

The records may be used as evidence to show that valid consent was obtained. They will be used to answer any allegation in respect of a civil claim for damages for trespass to the person or a criminal charge of assault and battery.

Records documenting consent should show that the health professional has discharged their duty of care. The records should demonstrate that they have properly informed the patient of the options and risks.

In particular, the health professional needs to consider how to document risks, any advice given and language barrier problems. Details of how to record risks and advice are set out below. To summarise, health professionals need to bear in mind the following points:

Risks

Detailed notes must be made of the risks about which the health professional has advised the patient. It is not enough to record simply 'advised of risks'.

If a dispute arises it will usually be in respect of the detail. The example given earlier was that the patient may say, 'Yes, you advised me of the risks. However, you said I might get an infection, but you did not tell me that I might bleed and had I known that I would not have had the operation'.

With the aid of the records the health professional will need to demonstrate the risks of which they actually advised the patient.

Failing to record the details of the risks about which the patient has been advised could mislead other health professionals involved in the patient's care.

EXAMPLE OF MISLEADING LACK OF DETAIL

A patient has been advised by the health professional of the usual risks of a surgical procedure and records 'patient advised of risks'.

The patient is visited by the anaesthetist prior to surgery. The anaesthetist may assume from the record that **all** of the risks have been explained to the patient, including not only the usual risks of that procedure, but also any other risk relating to the patient's underlying condition. For example, the patient may have a history of asthma. The anaesthetist may assume from the record that, in addition to the usual risks of the procedure, the risks in relation to the patient's asthma and the implications for general anaesthetic have also been explained to the patient. In reality no such additional risks have been explained to the patient.

The entry 'advised of risks' is misleading.

Remember, the records are for the benefit of the patient. The purpose of documenting the risks and advice is not defensive, that is to cover the health professional's back, but to ensure that all health professionals involved in the care of the patient are clear whether the patient has been fully informed.

Advice

Health professionals must set out in the notes the facts presented to the patient. Remember, it is not enough to write 'patient advised' in the records.

The notes should contain detail of the advice given, the risks and the options. If the patient refuses treatment or does not wish to accept the recommended treatment or advice, then such refusal should be clearly recorded. The patient may chose not to give a reason why they are refusing treatment (this is, after all, the patient's prerogative). However, the fact that the patient does not wish to give a reason should also be recorded.

It must be borne in mind that the health professional should be working in partnership with the patient. They may be able to explore the reasons why treatment is being refused and to reassure the patient, whilst at the same time respecting the patient's right of consent.

Details of leaflets given to the patient, including the name of those leaflets, should also be recorded.

Language and understanding

The health professional must have regard to the patient's understanding, which can be hampered by, for example, language, literacy barriers, mental health problems or confusion.

The health professionals should ask themselves:

➤ did the patient understand?

➤ how do you know they have understood?

➤ is the patient literate?

➤ do they need an interpreter?

Consider whether it is appropriate to have a family member as an interpreter. Will there be a risk of coercion if the family member exerts pressure or undue influence upon the patient?

Mental capacity

Consider whether there is an issue about the patient's mental capacity. If there is, record it in detail very carefully. Include in this detail how the patient's mental capacity was assessed.

Consent forms

The Department of Health has published 'Good Practice in Consent Implementation Guide'[4] and 'Consent Key Documents'.[5] These publications contain standard consent forms, which can be used or adapted by the Trusts or health professionals. There are four forms:

1 Patient agreement to investigation and treatment.
2 Patient agreement to investigation and treatment of a child or young person.
3 Patient/parental agreement to investigation and treatment (procedures where consciousness is not impaired).
4 Adults who are unable to consent to investigation and treatment.

Health professionals, when using the standard consent forms or where Trusts have adapted them for certain procedures, should take care when completing the forms to ensure that any additional information is recorded either on the forms themselves or in the health records (e.g. where the patient has an underlying condition such as diabetes or a heart problem). This will need to be taken into account and the documentation should reflect this.[4,5]

A careful record should be made of who signed the consent form if, for example, the patient is a child.

Remember also to apply the same best practice guidelines to the use of standard forms as discussed in Chapter 7.

Health professionals can read more detail about consent in the consent book in this series.

UNDERSTANDING, LANGUAGE AND INTERPRETERS

How do you know that the patient has understood what you have advised? Patients will often be passive and may not have the confidence to say they have failed to understand something. A good way of checking whether the patient has understood is to ask them to repeat it back to you in their own words.

If you give the patient a leaflet, how do you know they can read it? Is the patient literate? Patients who are illiterate are very clever at disguising it. They may not admit they are illiterate for fear of embarrassment.

If there is a language barrier, this should be clearly recorded. The health professional must ask themselves, 'Does the patient require an interpreter?' If an interpreter is used, record their name and ask the interpreter to countersign the record as having correctly interpreted the information.

If you are using a family member to interpret, you must be careful to use them appropriately and be aware of the confidentiality issues this raises. Health professionals must ask themselves, 'Is it appropriate to have a family member as interpreter? Is there a risk of coercion?' Failure to deal with these issues could invalidate consent and may also be a breach of confidentiality.

Where there are any issues regarding language and understanding then it is important to record the details.

DATES AND TIMES

All of the entries in the records should be dated and timed. This is evidence of a contemporaneous note.

Date

All entries should be fully dated. A common error in the record is failing to include the year, and simply writing, for example, 04/06. When it comes to reviewing records, omitting the year can create considerable confusion. The date in full should be included in all entries. The entry should be clear: the date the patient was seen and the date the entry was made (if it was made retrospectively). *See* the section on 'Retrospective entries' (page 87).

Time

The time of all entries should be recorded. Failure to record accurate timings can impact on clinical decisions and the absence of timings can be misleading. Timings help to provide a good clinical picture and provide the timeframe for assessing the progress of the patient or their deterioration.

Is there a common reference point for time? Is your watch synchronised with the clock on the ward or clock in theatre? Are the timings on the equipment synchronised? Are they altered when the clocks go forward and backwards?

EXAMPLE OF INCONSISTENT TIMINGS

In one case there was a six-minute discrepancy between the notes and the printout from equipment (a CTG machine). When asked, the writer of the notes explained: 'I always keep my watch six minutes fast, but sometimes I forget this when I'm writing my notes'!

In some areas of clinical practice, such as obstetric care, this lack of care in recording timings can have disastrous consequences. Six minutes can mean the difference in delivering a healthy baby or a brain-damaged baby. It can mean the life or death of a baby. Failure to record accurate timings can mean the difference between a claim for £5 million or no claim at all.

The recording of accurate timings is required, appropriate and essential in all healthcare settings.

There is sometimes confusion among health professionals about what timings should be recorded. Do we record time when we attended to the patient, or the time when we write up our entries?

The record should be clear and it should state the time you saw the patient. It should not state the time you should have seen the patient.

Take the following scenario, which occurs sometimes in community care.

EXAMPLE OF RECORDING TIMINGS

An appointment is in the diary for the health professional to see the patient at 10.30 hours. The health professional arrives at 11.00 hours. At the end of the day the health professional returns to the office arriving at 16.00 hours. They write up the records.

What time should be recorded in the entry: 10.30 hours, 11.00 hours or 16.00 hours?

There is no single way to record this. However, the entry in the records should be clear that the patient was seen at 11.00 hours. The time reflects the facts: the patient presented with a particular history and symptoms at a particular time. The entry in the record should state that it was actually written at 16.00 hours.

Imagine, for a moment, that the entry records the patient's temperature, but the entry is erroneously timed as 16:00 hours when the record was made instead of 11.00 hours when temperature was actually taken.

At 17.00 hours the patient is seen by another health professional. If the patient's condition deteriorates the health professional will not have an accurate account of the clinical picture and may make the wrong decision based upon it. This is because it would appear from the records that the change in the patient's temperature had only occurred in the previous hour (between 16.00 hours and 17.00 hours). In fact, these changes had occurred over the previous six hours (from 11.00 hours to 17.00 hours).

Inaccurately recorded timings are a common cause for a breakdown in communication in the records.

Some Trust policies state that the time the patient was seen should be written in the margin and the time the entry was recorded should be noted at the end of the entry or after the signature. (*See* the section on 'Retrospective entries' on page 87.)

How long?

It is sometimes appropriate to record the length of the consultation, meeting or patient contact.

This can be recorded by documenting the start time and finish time, (*see* example Record 1 below), or the time the consultation commenced and the length of time spent with the patient (*see* example Record 2 below).

Documenting the length of time the consultation or patient contact has taken demonstrates the level of care provided.

Consider this: a health professional attends the patient, they change the dressing, assist them with feeding, discuss the patient's planned care and give them advice. At a later date the patient alleges that the health professional merely popped their head around the door and that they neither discussed planned care nor gave advice.

TASK 7.1

Ask yourself:

Would the patient be believed if the consultation lasted for five minutes?

Would the health professional be believed if the consultation lasted for 1 hour and 10 minutes?

We can see from this scenario that it is more likely that the health professional will be believed where the consultation lasted for 1 hour and 10 minutes. The length of time spent with the patient reflects the level of care given (*see* Chapter 18, 'Health records used as evidence').

It may not be appropriate to record the length of time spent with patients in every circumstance; for example, in a high dependency unit where the patient is being constantly monitored. However, it can be useful in situations where there is a consultation between the patient and doctor, a care assessment or at a multidisciplinary meeting and so on.

Retrospective entries

If, for some reason, the health professional is prevented from making the contemporaneous note in the records they may make a retrospective entry. It is good practice to state when the entry was made and why the entry has been made retrospectively. For example, the health professional may have been called away on an emergency.

It is the practice of some health professionals when making a retrospective entry to note in the records the time the patient was actually seen, and under the signature to record the date and time that the entry was actually made.

EXAMPLE

Record 1

Date	Clinical notes (*each entry must be signed*)
12/06/05	The patient complained of feeling nauseas . . . .
16.30	*J. Smith*

Joanne Smith
SRN

13th June 2005 09.30 h

Another way of recording this is to set out clearly in the entry the time and date the patient was seen and the time the entry was made.

Record 2

Date	Clinical notes (*each entry must be signed*)
12/06/05	I saw the patient at 16.30 hours. She complained of feeling
16.30	Nauseas . . . .

I am writing this entry retrospectively on 13/06/05 at 09.30 h because I was called away on an emergency. *J. Smith*

Joanne Smith
SRN

It must be made clear when the patient was seen and, if the entry was made retrospectively, when that entry was made.

You should seek guidance at local level as to the preferred way to write retrospective entries.

AUTHENTICATE

Dr T Bolton   Dr Timothy Bolton
Specialist Registrar Paediatrics Pin 02098 (bleep 2345)

All entries in the records must be authenticated. It is essential that the author of the records is easily identifiable.

The Clinical Negligence Scheme for Trusts (CNST) Risk Management Standards 2005 suggests that when signing the records there should be a system in place which is clearly understood and used by all relevant staff. This could include name, personal identification numbers (PIN) or a central registry of sample signatures.[6]

The health professional should sign each entry. Their name must be printed alongside the entry, with the designation of the signatory. The professional registration or PIN number may also be recorded.

What is the purpose of authenticating the record?

One of the reasons for signing the entry in the record is because the writer is accountable for their entry. Another reason for authenticating and printing the name alongside the entry is so that the reader can clearly identify the writer in case they need to obtain more information about the patient. It is for this reason that a doctor will sometimes document their bleep number. This is very useful information to the health professionals. It saves a lot of time when the health professional is trying to locate the writer.

Whilst the use of a central registry of sample signatures is useful, often the signatures when reproduced do not appear as identical copies of those on the sample register. When the health professional is busy the signature may be rushed and may not resemble the sample. This causes a problem for health professionals who are relying upon those records if they need to contact the writer but cannot recognise the signature.

Who should sign the records?

The person who carries out the care and treatment should sign the entry in the record. This includes unregistered staff with first-hand knowledge of the care of the patient.

Countersigning the records

Countersigning might be required by registered staff in certain circumstances; for example, where members of staff are being supervised, such as students or healthcare assistants. In these circumstances, the supervisor might countersign the records. The purpose of countersigning is to ensure that the supervisor is satisfied that the treatment has been carried out competently. It does not necessarily indicate that the supervisor has witnessed the care carried out.

Countersigning gives the supervisor the opportunity to satisfy himself that the care was appropriate and to clarify any issues the entries raise. The supervisor may wish to add to the records where clarification is needed. The signatory and anyone who countersigns the records may be required to give evidence in respect of these records.

The health professional should confirm at local level what is required when authenticating and countersigning the records.

DESIGNATED PLACE FOR RECORDING ALLERGIES

In the records, there should be a designated place for recording allergies. It is important that this information is clearly visible and accessible to avoid a breakdown in communication.

Allergies recorded only in the body of a clinical or nursing entry could easily be overlooked. Use the designated documentation properly. The problems and breakdown in communication in respect of this are illustrated in the case study in Chapter 4.

It is essential too that health professionals read the documentation and act upon the allergy information it contains. Health professionals should look out for this information and they will need to know where to find it.

STANDARD FORMS AND TICK BOXES

There are often procedures in place to assist good record keeping. Standard forms can be very useful in maintaining good record keeping. They avoid the need for the health professional to have to write out the information in time-consuming longhand, can provide the health professional with very useful information and minimise the risk of omitting information by reminding them of the questions that need to be asked.

Where standard forms are implemented, they should be used properly. They are being used for good reason: they provide the health professional with information. However, there is often the temptation simply to pay lip service to them, as they are often incomplete. Standard forms are there to assist, so when they are being used they must be used properly.

Where there are forms with boxes to be ticked, fill in all the boxes and read each statement or comment to which the box refers.

What does an empty tick box mean? Does it mean it is not relevant, it has not been asked, or that the health professional needs to come back to it?

If it is not applicable then write that down, but never leave it blank. If it is left blank the court's view is that you did not even consider it and an adverse inference will be drawn.

Care plans

Standard forms, such as care plans, can lead to confusion if they are not properly completed. During the course of patient care, information may change. Such changes, including the time and dates of those changes, must be clearly recorded on the care plan.

It is not sufficient to amend the body of the care plan and then simply to re-sign and re-date the end of the document. Changes may occur several times during the care of the patient. If re-dates are only done at the end of the document, it may not be obvious to the reader when the changes took place.

It will be difficult for the health professional to follow the timescale of the progress or deterioration of the patient's condition. This is a particular problem with the mobility scores, for example. These scores will often change and will be amended, but with no indication as to when those changes occurred. This can result in changes, particularly subtle changes, in the patient's condition being overlooked.

LEGIBILITY

The records should be written clearly, legibly and in such a manner that they cannot be erased.

Health professionals should take care to ensure that their entries can be read by others. Sometimes there are difficulties when people can't even read their own writing! Often health professionals learn to read their own style of writing and that of their colleagues, but remember that the records may be read by others outside your department and Trust.

If a mistake is made because your writing is illegible, you will be accountable. If you cannot read the writing of another health professional, you should take steps to find out what it says. If you do not do this and you act on illegible records, you, as well as the writer, may be accountable.

The notes should preferably be written in black ink. The records will be shared with other health professionals and other disciplines, so they may need to be photocopied or faxed. The records need to be clear enough that they can be easily read when reproduced. Some coloured inks may not copy well.

The records should never be written in pencil. Fountain pen should be avoided as the ink can sometimes run if, for example, liquid is spilt on the records.

You should also have regard to guidelines set down by local policy and professional bodies. For example, pharmacists conventionally write in green ink.

REFERENCES

1 The Hazards of Diagnosing over the Telephone, 28/04/2005, Nick Gray – Alexander Harris solicitors. Article Available at: http://alexanderharris.co.uk/article/The_hazards_of_diagnosing_over_the_telephone_2343.asp#navigation

2 Department of Health, Health Service Commissioner. *Annual Report 2002–3* E.0410/00–1.

3 Royal College of Nursing. *Guidance for Nursing Practitioners: telephone advice lines for people with long term conditions*; 2006. Available at: www.rcn.org.uk/search?queries_search_query=telephone+advice+lines (accessed 11 February 2009).

4 Department of Health. *Good Practice in Consent Implementation Guide*; 2001. Available at: www.dh.gov.uk/en/AdvanceSearchResult/index.htm?searchTerms=consent+implementation+guide (accessed 11 February 2009).

5 The Department of Health. *Consent Key Documents*; 2004. Available at: www.dh.gov.uk/en/Publichealth/Scientificdevelopmentgeneticsandbioethics/Consent/Consentgeneralinformation/index.htm (accessed 11 February 2009).

6 Clinical Negligence Scheme for Trusts. *Risk Management Standards*; 2005. Available at: www.nhsla.com/Claims/Schemes/CNST/ (accessed 11 February 2009).

CHAPTER 8

Fact, assumption, professional opinion

It is important to distinguish between fact, assumption and professional opinion.

FACT AND ASSUMPTION

A fact can best be described as something that is known to have happened or to exist, especially something for which proof exists, or about which there is information. It is extremely important when making entries in the records that assumptions are **not** made. If assumptions are made there is a real danger that they will be recorded as if they were fact.

FIRST EXAMPLE OF AN ASSUMPTION

In a set of records a nurse recorded that 'the patient fell out of bed'.

The barrister asked the nurse in the witness box, 'Where were you standing at the time?'

She replied, 'I wasn't there at all'.

The barrister then asked, 'How do you know then that the patient fell out of bed?'

The nurse replied, 'I was at the nurses' station and on returning to the ward I found the patient on the floor'.

The barrister retorted, 'So you cannot say that the patient fell out of bed. That is an assumption'.

We use assumptions all the time in everyday life. At a job interview it is said that the interviewer will have made a decision within the first 30 seconds about whether the candidate is right for the job. The next half an hour of the interview is merely to clarify qualifications and experience and so on. However, when dealing with health records making assumptions is dangerous.

There is a danger that if we make an assumption it may be recorded as if it were a fact.

TASK 8.1

'The patient was drunk'

List ways in which a patient might present if they were drunk?

The patient may present as confused, aggressive, have slurred speech, be incoherent, and be unsteady on their feet.

How many conditions might these symptoms indicate? There are many conditions that may account for these symptoms, such as stroke, dementia, or a brain tumour. If we make an assumption that the patient was drunk based on the presenting symptoms, then we may mistake the true nature of the patient's condition.

The danger of recording 'the patient was drunk' is a problem because the lack of detail of the patient's presenting symptoms may lead to a failure to recognise the patient's true condition and so fail to diagnose and treat the patient appropriately.

SECOND EXAMPLE OF AN ASSUMPTION

A patient who was suffering from diabetes was out shopping in a supermarket for a bottle of wine for his dinner guests. At the checkout he collapsed and the bottle broke, causing the contents to spill over his coat. He was taken to hospital by ambulance. He was confused, incoherent and smelling of alcohol. An assumption was made that the patient was drunk. As result there was failure to diagnose that his symptoms were due to diabetes. The patient died.

Remember too that the rationale must be recorded. How did we reach the conclusion that the patient was drunk?

We could record in the records that 'the patient presented as confused, had slurred speech, unsteady gait and was incoherent. The patient appeared to be drunk'.

If it is recorded in this factual way it is more likely that the correct treatment will be provided. If the facts and the timings are recorded, then if the patient deteriorates it will be clear from the notes that it is unlikely to be as a result of the alcohol because the symptoms would usually diminish as the effects of the alcohol wear off. Therefore, if the symptoms continue or get worse it is likely that there is another cause. But in the absence of facts about how the patient presented it will be impossible to measure if the symptoms have changed and if the patient is deteriorating.

Other common assumptions are 'the patient appears to be in pain'. What should be recorded is that the 'patient states that they are in pain'.

Maternity notes sometimes report that 'pain is under control'. Perhaps if we were to ask the mother in labour whether the pain is under control then she might take a different view!

Another common assumption is an entry which reads 'the patient was depressed'. Are we qualified to make this diagnosis? We should record the facts. For example:

➤ 'the patient presented as tearful'
➤ 'she states she has not eaten for several days and is not sleeping more than two hours a night'
➤ 'she says she is not getting any support from her family'
➤ 'the patient said she was in a low mood'.

Read the following paragraph and then consider the statements below.

TASK 8.2

Kim Smith had an appointment for admission into the surgical ward on 4 October 2006. The consultant, Dr Roberts, had recommended that the patient undergo a colonoscopy. Following a procedure the patient complained that she was in pain. Dr Roberts suggested that Smith be referred for genetic testing. The patient was discharged and an appointment was given for six weeks later.

Which is fact and which assumption?

	Fact	Assumption
1 Mrs Smith was admitted on 4 October 2006		
2 The patient was seen by Dr Roberts		
3 The patient underwent a colonoscopy		
4 The patient was given pain relief		
5 The patient was referred for genetic testing		
6 The patient attended the hospital six weeks later.		

These are all assumptions.

1 **Mrs** Smith is an assumption. It states **Kim** Smith – we do not know the gender or whether the patient was married. The statement records that Kim Smith had an 'appointment for admission', not that she was admitted.
2 The consultant Dr Roberts recommended a colonoscopy. The patient was not necessarily seen by Dr Roberts.
3 The patient was admitted for colonoscopy but it does not say that it was carried out.
4 The patient was in pain. It does not state that the patient was given pain relief.
5 It was suggested by Dr Roberts that the patient be referred for genetic testing. It does not state that she was actually referred.
6 The patient was given an appointment for six weeks later. It does not state that she attended six weeks later.

The danger of making assumptions is that something is likely to be overlooked. For example, it may be assumed that the patient has been referred for genetic testing when actually nothing more has happened.

PROFESSIONAL OPINION

An assumption is quite different from a professional opinion. As a health professional it is your role to assess the needs of the patient, to diagnose or decide upon the care or treatment. When the patient presents, the health professional takes a history, finds out about symptoms, notes the signs and forms an opinion about what the patient requires in terms of treatment, care, medication or referral to a specialist or GP. It is quite proper then for a health professional to form a professional opinion based upon the facts and this is very different from making an assumption.

CHAPTER 9

Amending the records

From time to time it may be necessary to correct an error or mistake in the records. These are the only circumstances where amendments can take place.

When amending the records you should score out the error with a single line, which should then be signed and timed and dated by the person who has made the amendment.

Erasers, liquid paper (like Tippex) or any other obliterating agents should never be used to cancel errors.

The original entry underneath must be clear to read. You should never scribble out the original entry so that it cannot be read. The court will think you are hiding something.

Remember that the record is a tool for communicating. It should be evident to the reader why the amendment was necessary. For example, an erroneous entry may state that the patient has diabetes when they do not because the entry has been written in the wrong patient's notes. In addition to amending the record in the appropriate way, it would also be prudent to write the reason for the error to make sure that the correct information is communicated.

AMENDING MENTAL HEALTH RECORDS

Where the records relate to the detention and treatment of those with mental health problems, correction of records may only be made in certain circumstances, which are set out in the Mental Health Act 1983.[1] The documents are the legal basis for detention and a health professional who fails to adhere to the provisions of the Act may be committing an offence, as could anyone who permits the use of such documents. Errors can be amended, but only in specific circumstances pursuant to Section 15.[2]

Errors that can be amended include:

➤ leaving blank any of the spaces on the form
➤ failure to delete one or more alternatives
➤ patient's forename and surname not agreeing in different places on documents
➤ neither of the doctors providing the medical recommendation being approved under Section 12.[3]

Examples of situations where there can be no amendment are:

If the application is fundamentally flawed – this was the ruling by the Court of Appeal in the case of Re S-C.[4] The court held that rectification of the records cannot be used to cure a defect, which is a fundamental flaw in the process leading to detention. In other words, you cannot amend the records to show what should have been done, rather than what was actually done.

The case of R v South Western Hospital Managers 1994[5] – it was held that rectification is concerned with the correction of errors on the face of the document, such as:

➤ if there is no signature
➤ if the medical recommendations do not include a specific form of mental disorder
➤ if the statutory time limits are exceeded
➤ if a signatory is not empowered to be such under the Act (e.g. the doctor is excluded under Section 12; the social worker is not approved; where the applicant purports to be the nearest relative, but the signatory is not in fact the nearest relative as defined in the Act)
➤ If 14 days have elapsed since the patient was admitted.

Health professionals working in mental health must make themselves familiar with the relevant legislation.

REFERENCES

1 The Mental Health Act 1983.
2 The Mental Health Act 1983, S15.
3 The Mental Health Act 1983, S12.
4 Re S-C (Mental Patient: Habeas Corpus) 1996 1 All ER 532 CA.
5 R v South Western Hospital Managers, ex p. M 1994 1 All ER 161.

CHAPTER 10

What to leave out

JARGON

The Cambridge English Dictionary defines jargon as: 'Special words and phrases which are used by particular groups of people, especially in their work'.

The NMC Guidelines state that jargon should not be included in the records.[1] Jargon may not be understood by others who may rely on the records; for example, the patient, carers, other health professionals or other agencies, such as social services.

In the HSC Annual Report for 2003–4 the HSC stated that some of the complaints investigated might never have arisen if health professionals had communicated clearly with patients without using jargon, had taken the time to ensure that patients and carers understood what was being said to them and had made a record of the conversation.[2]

Poor communication accounts for a large number of complaints. Jargon can hamper communication and result in complaints – or worse, it can impact negatively on patient care.

ROUTINE AND MEANINGLESS ENTRIES

If writing the records is delayed, and if there is lack of detail, there is a danger that records will become routine and meaningless. They will move away from their real purpose, which is to facilitate treatment, care and support of the patient.

In an article by Bridgit Dimond, Barrister and author, she states:

> 'Records should be a meaningful and clear account of the patients' care. "Had a good day", which is one of the most unhelpful statements, should not feature in the records. Why did she have a good day? Had her appetite returned? Had she spent most of the time sleeping? Alternatively, had she spent most of the day awake? Had she been of minimal trouble to the nursing staff? Had she in contrast been lively and interacted with the nursing staff? All of these situations, many of them incompatible, are within the meaning of those words'.[3]

TASK 10.1

Following a night shift, you pick up 15 sets of records.
What will they read?

It is not uncommon to see in each set of records the same entry, which reads along the lines of, 'patient slept well'.

If you ask the patient if they slept well, what will they say? Their answer will probably be, 'I didn't sleep at all'.

Staff on the night shift will say 'I was rushed off my feet'. How come, when all of the patients were sleeping?

These are routine and meaningless entries. They do not reflect the care that has really been provided for the patient. They lead to a breakdown in communication and compromise patient care.

During the night shift, the patient will have been observed, their pulse taken and so on. This should be recorded. It can be extremely useful for the doctor the next morning on his ward round to know what the patient's pulse rate was during the previous night.

There have been entries in the records which state 'patient slept well', when the patient had actually been dead for several hours.

It was reported in *The Times* that in one set of patient notes it was recorded:

'6:30am sleeping peacefully
8:40am dead'[4]

You must write in the records what actually happened and not what ought to have happened or what you would 'usually do'. Health professionals are often involved in carrying out similar procedures with patients who have similar conditions and thus there is a danger that the facts relating to each patient can be confused. In these circumstances, you should exercise caution to ensure that the detail in the record reflects the care provided for each patient. For example, if you are working in the diabetic clinic you would usually ask each patient the same questions; you give them the same advice, the same leaflets and may record this almost identically in each record.

However, sometimes there are distractions – perhaps because the patient had asked a question, or maybe the leaflet usually given had run out.

Sometimes, because the procedure and advice is routine, we may assume that we have informed the patient when in fact we have not, but because our entries are routine they may then reflect what we **should have done** and **not what we actually did**.

It is vital to record what we actually did.

GRATUITOUS ENTRIES

We often see gratuitous entries in the records. An example of this is 'lovely child'. Another example in a health visitor record is an entry which reads 'tatty house and garden'. What does this mean? Perhaps that the patient does not have the latest designer curtains! This is a subjective comment and a gratuitous entry. What is the health visitor trying to convey? Possibly the health professional is concerned about risk. Maybe they are concerned that somebody is not coping or there is a risk to a child or a vulnerable adult. But how do we know what that risk is? How do we measure the risk? How do we plan the care? How do we know if any planned care put in place is effective if we have nothing to measure it by?

These kinds of entries do not assist with patient care and have no place in the records. If we are concerned about risk then we should be explicit and record the facts. If it is not recorded in this way then something will be missed and patients will be placed at risk.

These kinds of entries should be avoided as they add nothing and do not assist with patient care, treatment or support.

SUBJECTIVE COMMENTS

A subjective comment is influenced by or based on personal beliefs or feelings, rather than facts. The NMC Guidelines state that the records should not include 'irrelevant speculation and offensive subjective statements'.[5]

An offensive subjective comment may be, for example, 'Dull as a door stop'. This kind of entry is offensive, subjective and unprofessional.

Such comments should not be written in the records.

ABBREVIATIONS

The NMC guidelines state that abbreviations should not be used in the records.[6] Abbreviations cause a lot of confusion and can lead to the patient's care being compromised, as there is a risk that the abbreviation will be misunderstood. Such a misunderstanding may result in the patient being given the wrong treatment, medication or care.

If a patient is harmed as a result of the use of abbreviations, the writer of the record will be accountable. The reader who relied upon it may also be accountable.

Many abbreviations have more than one meaning so it is difficult for those caring for the patient to ascertain the intended meaning. Remember, care is shared amongst a number of health professionals. Your records will be read by junior staff, agency staff, locums, health professionals in different disciplines and those new to the Trust or the field of practice. They may not be familiar with or understand the abbreviation or they may misinterpret it and give it a different meaning.

The meaning of abbreviations varies between different Trusts, and even between departments in the same Trust. Abbreviations lack clarity and could be ambiguous.

For example, the abbreviation DOA may mean 'Dead on Arrival' but can also be confused with 'Date of Admission'. You can see the difficulties this may cause. Although one would hope that the health professional would appreciate the difference when the patient presents!

Common examples of ambiguous abbreviations include:
➤ FBC: full blood count *or* fluid balance chart
➤ P/T: part time *or* physiotherapist *or* patient
➤ OD: once daily *or* overdose
➤ HV: health visitor *or* home visit

➤ CHD: chronic heart disease *or* congenital heart disease *or* congenital hip dysphasia
➤ SC: subcutaneous *or* self caring
➤ DNR: do not resuscitate *or* district nurse referral
➤ Px: patient *or* prescribed
➤ Dx: diagnosed *or* discharged
➤ BG: blood glucose *or* blood gas(es)
➤ BM: bone marrow *or* blood monitoring
➤ Ca: calcium *or* cancer *or* carcinoma
➤ CT: chemotherapy *or* CT scan
➤ MM: millimole *or* millimetre *or* malignant melanoma
➤ pH: hydrogen potential *or* past history.

In one set of records the abbreviation used was FLK which is short for 'Funny Looking Kid'. This is an abbreviation sometimes seen in obstetric or midwifery records. The reason for FLK is that perhaps the newborn infant's appearance causes the health professionals concern about their potential development, but tests do not reveal anything concrete. The health professional will usually wish to review the infant in, say, six weeks to see if the infant is progessing normally. In a set of records, the entry 'FLK review six weeks' was made and on the six-week entry it read, 'It's ok, we've seen the father'. This is very embarrassing and not something you would want to have to explain in the witness box!

Best practice dictates that abbreviations should not be used. However, it has been suggested that this is impractical and that departments should have lists of approved abbreviations that are also made available to patients so that they understand what they mean.

It is often the practice that members of staff are issued with the list of abbreviations or the list is in a conspicuous place on the ward. However, this will not assist the reader who is in another department, from a different discipline, or from an outside agency, such as social services.

A list of approved abbreviations will not eliminate the risk of misunderstanding, but it will reduce the risk. Lists of abbreviations should ideally be placed with each set of records so that the user of the records has a quick reference point.

Any list of abbreviations should be kept to a minimum and must be approved by the Trust, employer or organisation. Don't be tempted to add your own abbreviations to the list.

ARROWS AND DASHES

Do not use arrows and dashes in the records; longhand should be used. These are only understood by the writer and after time not even by them. Arrows and dashes do not clearly explain their meaning and can lead to confusion and therefore will compromise patient care.

DO NOT SQUEEZE INFORMATION IN

Do not try to squeeze information into the entry in the records. You should not insert information with an arrow as shown below.

EXAMPLE OF INSERT

In a set of maternity records the entry read:

       loose
'cord∧around baby's neck'

You can see the adverse connotation this may have.

If you have left something out of the record then you should amend it in the appropriate way (*see* page 99) or write it up retrospectively and explain why (*see* page 87).

DO NOT LEAVE GAPS

Do not be tempted to leave gaps in the records. If, for example, you know that your colleague has seen the patient, but has not yet written up their entry in the record, do not leave a gap in the record for your colleague to fill in later. When you see the patient you will have acted on the information you had at that time.

What would happen if, after you have seen the patient, your colleague makes an entry in the gap in the record, and that entry contains information that would have changed the way in which you had treated the patient?

For example, after you treat the patient your colleague makes a retrospective entry in the gap in the record: 'Rang lab and test results confirm diabetes'. You did not have this information at the time you saw the patient and you may have commenced the wrong treatment or given something that is contraindicated due to the diabetes. At the time you saw the patient you acted appropriately on the information you had at that time.

What will the court think?

When something goes wrong the fault may take days, weeks or months to come to light. If, sometime later, you were asked to review your notes and explain what happened, you might look at those notes and wonder, 'What was I thinking giving that medication when the patient had diabetes?' Or you may actually remember, 'This is the day when I left a gap in the records, and I therefore did not have that information when I saw the patient'. Looking at the records do you think you would persuade the court that is what happened? It is highly unlikely that the court would be persuaded.

This raises another, more important issue. The failure to write the contemporaneous note results in a breakdown of communication. There is a danger that as the information has been written up in the gap in the record, it will be missed. It is more likely to be overlooked. This compromises patient care and also exposes the health professionals to legal and professional consequences.

If it is necessary to leave a blank line in the records to distinguish one entry from another, then you should put a diagonal line through it.

If there are, say, two or three lines left at the bottom of the page, but you wish to start a new page, you should put a diagonal line through the blank spaces. There is nothing more frustrating than commencing your entry at the bottom of the page and on turning over the page you find that the previous health professional had started a new page.

You should have regard to and adhere to local policy. Some Trusts do not allow any blank spaces.

REFERENCES

1 The Nursing and Midwifery Council. *Guidelines for Records and Record Keeping*; 2005. Available at: www.nmc-uk.org/aFrameDisplay.aspx?DocumentID=4008 (accessed 10 February 2009).
2 Department of Health, Health Service Commissioner. *Annual Report 2003–4*. E.2193/01–2.
3 Dimond B. Common deficiencies in record keeping. *Br J Nurs*. 2005; **14**(10): 568–70.
4 Wright O. Doctors taught art of writing patient notes. *The Times*. 9 June 2003.
5 The Nursing and Midwifery Council, op. cit.
6 Ibid.

CHAPTER 11

Common errors in the records

Investigations into complaints have revealed common errors in records which hampered the care provided or made it difficult for health professionals to defend their practice.

A consultant orthopaedic surgeon wrote to *The Times* in 2003. He stated that he had reviewed the records of 300 patients over 15 years for the purpose of medico-legal reports and found that 90% of the records were deficient. Prominent features were:

➤ failure to record an accurate history
➤ lack of an appropriate clinical examination
➤ operation notes that fail to record the findings
➤ operation notes that omit details of the procedure undertaken and complications that arise
➤ failure to record unexpected clinical developments, such as the onset of severe pain or limb paralysis
➤ illegibility including illegibility of the signature
➤ failure to record information given by the doctor to the patient before consent is obtained.

The surgeon considered that these defects had a significant impact on the conduct and outcome of medico-legal cases, especially in clinical negligence. He made the point that judges and lawyers generally would be uncompromising and robust when deciding on the significance of deficient records, which reflect and impact upon the standard of care. For example, if a clinical examination is not recorded, it must be assumed that it did not take place.[1]

Bridgit Dimond stated in an article that deficiencies were identified in a project on hospital-acquired infection.[2]

The project was undertaken by the Central Pathology Services at Collingwood in conjunction with selected NHS Trusts across the UK to identify the levels of hospital-acquired infection. They used hospital records to obtain data on levels of infection. However, they were thwarted by defects in the records. These defects included:

➤ no record of infection
➤ infection site not inspected
➤ meaningless entries such as the patient 'had a good day'
➤ defective care plan
➤ no signature
➤ no temperature or blood pressure recorded
➤ patient discomfort not recorded
➤ no record of any action
➤ no timings
➤ use of Tippex
➤ failure to list details involving invasive procedures: such as the date, inserted by? Type of device? Why was it used? When it was removed?
➤ antibiotics prescribed with no reason given or start or stop dates
➤ illegible handwriting
➤ value of pre-printed plans were lost as they were not completed.

Common errors in the records collated from a group of health visitors included:

➤ times omitted
➤ lack of entry in the record when an abortive call has been made
➤ illegible handwriting
➤ ambiguous abbreviations
➤ no record of phone call or name of the recipient
➤ use of Tippex and covering up of errors
➤ no signatures
➤ absence of information
➤ inaccuracies
➤ wrong dates
➤ omission of dates of medical checkups, hearing tests and immunisations
➤ record completed by someone who did not make the visit
➤ inaccuracies in name, date of birth, address

➤ unprofessional terminology
➤ meaningless phrases
➤ delay in completing the records, with sometimes more than 24 hours elapsing
➤ opinion mixed with fact
➤ reliance on information from neighbours with no identification of the source
➤ subjective comments.

TRANSMITTING AND RECEIVING INFORMATION

Record keeping should not be a chore but a positive tool for the care of the patient and a means of transmitting and receiving information.

In general, health professionals are good at transmitting information, but some are not so good at receiving it and, therefore, acting upon it.

EXAMPLE OF NOT ACTING ON INFORMATION RECEIVED

In one case, a nurse meticulously wrote up the patient's temperature, which was dangerously high. The nurse continued to write the notes, but did not take action.

I have seen many cases where test results are not acted upon. For example, in a CTG trace in obstetric care where it was even noted on the printout that it was a suspicious trace, no action was taken.

There is little point in writing up the notes if they are not read or acted upon. The records are a tool for communicating so do not just write them, but read and act upon them as well.

DUPLICATION OF HEALTH RECORDS

In some instances the records are duplicated several times. This is not uncommon in community care. For example, an entry is made in the patient-held record. An entry is then made in the professional's diary or notebook as an aide-memoire, then back at the office an entry is made in the main record and a further record is made to send to another agency, such as social services.

The entries should be made in all relevant records. The problem with this duplication is that there is a danger that there will be inconsistencies between the records. The more they are duplicated, the more room there is for error. If the matter were then to come to court the health professional would be vulnerable when giving evidence. The court will look for errors and inconsistencies between the records.

Duplication of records occurs both in community care and acute care. This process of duplication is very time consuming. How long does it take to write these records? It is not uncommon that several hours will be added to the end of the day in order to write them. This can feel like an onerous task to health professionals.

Some Primary Care Trusts (PCTs) have a system of recording in carbon copy form so that the information is written only once and the copies are placed in the relevant files. These systems free up the health professional's time. This is important when we know the time pressures on health professionals. This also avoids inconsistencies between the records.

Some PCTs provide staff with handheld computers known as PDAs (Personal Digital Assistants). The health professional can enter the information onto the PDA and then simply use the data or memory stick to transfer the information onto other computers. This avoids the need to retype the information.

In the Acute Trust, errors and inconsistencies can occur if rewriting nursing notes into the clinical notes. This should be avoided. The minute you start duplicating the records, there is room for error.

The case study in chapert 4 provides a good illustration of what can happen when transposing information between records. You will recall that the nurse erroneously left out part of an entry resulting in the abrupt withdrawal of a steroid, which caused the patient's death.

In some Acute Trusts they no longer have several records held by different departments, but use a single record instead. This avoids the need to duplicate the records. All health professionals attending the patient will make their entry in the same single record. This can be invaluable as it avoids any confusion about whether the patient has been seen by other health professionals and what the outcome is.

There is an obligation to copy letters to the patient. This is discussed in detail in Chapter 13. When copying letters to the patient or to the GP be careful that there are no inconsistencies between the records and the letters.

REFERENCES

1 Harris NH. Letter to the Editor: medical note taking. *The Times*. 18 June 2003.
2 Dimond B. Exploring common deficiencies that occur in record keeping. *Br J Nurs*. 2005; **14**(10): 568–70.

CHAPTER 12

Sharing information

The purpose of the records is to provide care for the patient; they are an effective tool to communicate this. However, the patient has the right to confidentiality and health professionals have a duty to uphold that right. Therefore, consent from the patient to disclose information should be sought. Whilst the health professional must uphold the patient's right of confidentiality they cannot guarantee it absolutely. This is because there are certain circumstances where it may be justifiable to breach confidentiality, and other circumstances where there is a statutory duty to breach it.

Where matters involve children or vulnerable adults, there is a duty that agencies cooperate in the sharing of records. There should be protocols in place for sharing information with other agencies.

INTER-PROFESSIONAL ACCESS TO RECORDS

The principle of shared records is that all members of the healthcare team involved in the care and treatment of an individual should make entries in a single record and in accordance with an agreed local protocol. The ability to obtain information whilst respecting patient and client confidentiality is essential.

Each health professional's contribution to such records should be seen as being of equal importance. This reflects the wider value of collaborative working within the inter-professional healthcare team.

The same right of access to records by the patient or client exists where a system of shared records is in use. It is essential, therefore, that local agreement is reached to identify and publicise who is responsible for considering requests from patients and clients for access in particular circumstances.

It is important that health professionals understand confidentiality so that the above can be put into context. Confidentiality is discussed briefly on page 121.

COMMUNICATION BETWEEN HEALTHCARE PROFESSIONALS

Good communication is an essential part of good clinical treatment. The records provide the tool for communication between health professionals. One of the difficulties for health professionals is making sense of a patient's condition and history where the records are contained in numerous documents.

Often the patient's records are fragmented. They may consist of, for example, the patient-held record, health visitor record, mental health record, GP and hospital records. This can be particularly problematic in community care. The Acute Trusts are no strangers to fragmented records. The records consist of, for example, the nursing notes, clinical notes, physiotherapy notes, occupational therapy notes and so on. The more fragmented the records the more room there is for a breakdown of communication. There must be systems in place for the sharing of information.

Pharmacists may now prescribe medication, as well as dispense it, under the rules of non-medical prescribing. The cornerstone of non-medical prescribing is good record keeping. Particular attention must be paid to the Clinical Management Plan. The prescriber must have access to the patient's records, but how does the pharmacist access the records in practice? There must be a system in place for the pharmacist to access the patient records.

It is not a defence to treat a patient in the absence of full information simply because the full records were not to hand. For example, it would be foolish for a physiotherapist to say, 'I didn't know about the patient's fracture because I did not have the x-ray or the clinical notes to hand'.

Where a doctor or nurse does not have the records available when treating the patient because it takes three days for the records department to locate them, they will be accountable if that treatment is contraindicated. So what should they do?

The real danger is that the patient may be treated inappropriately. If the records are unavailable something will inevitably be missed.

EXAMPLE OF UNAVAILABLE RECORDS

In the HSC Annual Report 2002,[1] there is reference to a complaint following the death of a patient who had been admitted to hospital after a fall that led to fractures of the knee and pelvis. When the patient returned to the hospital for a routine fracture clinic appointment, the clinical note recorded that her left knee was displaced, but this note was not typed into the clinical records until some days later. No written instructions on the management of her knee were given when she returned the same day to a second hospital. She subsequently died in the second hospital after a septic knee had been diagnosed.

In this example, there was a lack of communication between the doctors, there was no formal structure for consultant cover, the level of documentation in the clinical notes was poor and the system of transferring information between hospitals in the Trust was not being adhered to, despite assurances to the contrary. Due to poor communications and lack of support for junior medical staff, opportunities were missed to tackle the sepsis spreading from her injuries.

How far do you need to go to locate the records before treating the patient?

In an emergency, the health professional may have little choice but to treat the patient on the basis of the information they have at the time.

In the normal course of events, if the patient's care is compromised because the health professional did not have the records to hand when treating the patient, it is not a defence for the health professional to say 'the records were not to hand at the time I saw the patient'.

How does the health professional manage the unavailability of records in practice?

Where, for example, a health visitor requires the GP's or other records, it is not enough to simply write to the GP for the records and, if they are not received, do nothing. It would be prudent for the health visitor to call the GP and to chase the records. Each contact or step taken to obtain the records should be meticulously recorded in the notes.

The court would certainly wish to know what measures were taken to obtain the information. More importantly, to treat the patient without the benefit of the records carries with it the risk of failing to treat the patient appropriately.

Fax and email communication

Fax communication must be dealt with carefully. It is not enough simply to send a fax. How does the health professional know that a fax has been received by the intended recipient? There may a transmission error or the ink in the fax printer at the other end may have dried up.

One way of dealing with faxes is to ask the recipient to acknowledge receipt or to call them a few minutes after the document is faxed to make sure they received it.

Caution must be exercised to ensure that the correct fax number has been used. A common mistake is made during weekends or out of office hours when often alternative out of hours fax numbers are used.

CASE STUDY

On 16 December 1997 *The Times* reported that a girl died because her medical records were faxed to a machine in a locked room to which no-one had access over the weekend.[2] The girl was aged five years and suffered from giant cell hepatitis. She fell ill on a visit to Middlesbrough, where, in ignorance of her medical history, she was given a new drug, Tacrolimus, and suffered a massive overdose.

Health professionals must be aware of the issues of confidentiality where the location of the recipient's fax machine may be in a common area where documents received may be seen by someone other than the intended recipient.

Further consideration should be given to faxing documents between authorities relating to the detention of mental health patients. In order to ensure that there can be no confusion or room for error, health professionals should not rely solely on a faxed document.

As the document is the basis of the justification of the patient's detention, there should be additional precautions to ensure the validity of a detention based on faxed documents. Thus Richard Jones suggests that the recipient should confer with the signatory by telephone to confirm that the form was completed by the signatory and that the original form is delivered to the recipient at the earliest opportunity.[3]

Approved social workers should follow a similar procedure in making an application for detention in relation to the medical recommendations. The Home Office sometimes faxes documents to hospitals, but the hospital should insist that they receive the original documents as soon as possible. Similar provisions should take place when patients are transferred between hospitals. The receiving hospital should have the original documents relating to the patient's detention. The Mental Health Act Commission in its sixth Biennial Report endorsed the use of faxed forms.[4]

Similar precautions about checking with signatories would apply to documents that are scanned and sent by email to the recipient. The original documents should be forwarded as soon as possible.[5]

CONFIDENTIAL INFORMATION

One of the difficulties health professionals encounter with communication is the issue of confidentiality. Whilst health professionals must respect the patient's right to confidentiality, this should be dealt with in a way that does not breach their rights nor hinder communication between health professionals.

Health professionals must maintain a balance between providing quality care and preserving patient confidentiality.

Confidentiality is simple: don't say anything to anyone! The difficulty for the health professional is knowing when confidentiality can be justifiably breached. The health professional must be aware of and uphold the legal rights of patients in respect of confidentiality and should be aware of how to deal with the issues of confidentiality.

With regard to documentation and confidentiality, what do you do if the patient says to you, 'I am going to tell you something, but I do not want you to write it down and I do not want you to say anything'?

EXAMPLE

A child with a terminal illness was visited at home by a health visitor. The health visitor would usually make an entry in the patient-held record during the visit. The father of the child was a known drug user.

During the visit the child told the health visitor, 'I am going to tell you some-thing but I don't want you to tell my father and I don't want you to record it, but my father is stealing my morphine and using it for himself'.

The health visitor, not knowing how to deal with the documentation, pretended she had not heard it! The dilemma she faced was that if she had recorded it in the patient-held record, she may have placed the child at risk. She did not want to write it in the record because the child had told her not to, and she was worried about breaching confidentiality.

This is clearly unacceptable and raises the issue of duty of care that the child is now left without treatment. To have pretended she had not heard it is a breach of professional conduct. The health professional has an obligation to make a record.

There are practical and appropriate solutions to this scenario. Firstly, of course, the health visitor should have ensured that the child received the appropriate treatment and care. The health visitor could have arranged for a health professional to administer the medication regularly rather than leav-ing the drug in the home for self or parental administration.

As far as the documentation is concerned, it is important that all health professionals know the facts in a case in order to implement appropriate care. Because the entry in the patient-held records might have exposed the child to a risk, a supplementary record could have been implemented. (*See* further information in Chapter 14 on 'supplementary records'.)

If a patient tells you something and then asks you not to record it, you must still record it in the notes. Once the patient has told you something you cannot disregard it; you must record it. You have a professional obliga-tion to do so.

If the patient tells you 'I am going to tell you something but I don't want you to record it', you should inform them that you have an obligation to record what they tell you in the records. It is then up to the patient whether they tell you or not.

Health professionals working within the NHS can refer to the pub-lished consultation on the NHS code of practice regarding health records management.[6]

Can non-professionals record information?

In organisations where busy clinicians use dictation to record information, the organisation must ensure that non-health professionals, such as secretaries and receptionists who have access to confidential information, keep such information secure. The Royal College of Nursing (RCN) believes that until such time as fully reliable speech recognition software is available, then the practice of using non-professional staff will continue.

While it may be the case that asking a non-healthcare professional to input data onto electronic care records may put the confidentiality of records at risk (but that should be addressed by terms of employment of the receptionist as is the case with medical secretaries), it also has the potential to affect the accuracy of the record. However, best practice is for the 'treating clinician' to input data themselves and thus avoid mistakes in transcribing by a third party.[7]

It is important that the health professional fully understands patient confidentiality to ensure a complete understanding of the difference between the obligations to record information and in the circumstances in which that information can be shared with others and who those others might be.

Confidentiality is not covered in any depth in this book; nevertheless, health professionals must be aware of their legal and professional obligations in respect of it.

RECORDS USED FOR RESEARCH AND TEACHING

Patient records may be used for research, teaching purposes and clinical supervision. The patient should be informed and consent obtained to use the records for such purposes. The patient should also be informed that their refusal will not impact on their care. The principles of access and confidentiality remain the same and the right of the patient or client to refuse access to their records for this purpose should be respected.

The use of patient records in research should be approved by the local research ethics committee.

RECORDS USED FOR CLINICAL AUDIT

An audit is part of the risk management process. The aim is to promote high standards of care. If risks are identified and improvements made in healthcare, risks to patients and employees are minimised and the costs to the employer are reduced.

Audits may be made internally or by external regulatory bodies. Best practice in record keeping is a vital part of risk management and can assist in the audit process.

Where records are used for clinical audit then such an audit should be carried out by health professionals with clear professional obligations to maintain confidentiality. It is good ethical practice to take steps to inform patients that the quality of care is reviewed through the process of audit and that this might involve looking through a patient's records to produce anonymous audit data. If patients refuse to allow their information to be used for audit purposes, this should be respected and they should be informed that such refusal will not affect their treatment and care.

Increasingly, hospitals, Trusts and GP surgeries commission health professionals and commercial agencies to carry out audits on their behalf. In these circumstances, there must be a firm contractual and professional obligation to preserve confidentiality.

REFERENCES

1 Department of Health, Health Service Commissioner. *Annual Report 2002–3* E.0410/00–1.
2 News in Brief. Girl died after fax error at hospital. *The Times*. 16 December 1997.
3 Jones R. *Mental Health Act Manual*. 8th ed. London: Sweet and Maxwell; 2003.
4 Mental Health Act Commission. *Sixth Biennial Report 1993–1995*. Nottingham; Mental Health Act Commission; 1996.
5 Dimond B. Mental health records. *Br J Nurs*. 2005; **14**(21): 1132–4.
6 National Health Service. *Code of Practice: records management*. Available at: www.dh.gov. uk/en/Managingyourorganisation/Informationpolicy/Recordsmanagement/index.htm (accessed 11 February 2009).
7 Royal College of Nursing. *Record keeping in general practice: guidance on confidential patient information*. Available at: www.rcn.org.uk/development/communities/specialisms/ primary_care_and_public_health/forums/practice_nurses_association/record_keeping_in_ general_practice (accessed 11 February 2009).

CHAPTER 13

Access to health records by the patient

PATIENT'S RIGHT OF ACCESS TO HEALTH RECORDS

A patient is entitled to see personal information held about them. They are entitled to access to their health records. 'Health records' include all records relating to the patient's health.

The Data Protection Act 1998[1] governs access to health records. It gives the statutory right to a subject (i.e. the patient) to have access to their health records. The Act applies to computer and manual records. The Data Protection Act 1998 replaces the Data Protection Act 1984[2] and Access to Health Records Act 1990[3] (except in respect of records of deceased patients, where the Access to Health Records Act 1990 still applies).

The Data Protection Act 1998 applies not only to the NHS but also to the private health sector and to the private practice health records. It also applies to the records of employers who hold information relating to the physical or mental health of their employees, if the record has been made by or on behalf of a health professional in connection with the care of the employee.

The Act enables a patient to be:
- informed whether personal data is processed
- given a description of the data held, the purpose for which it is processed and to whom the data has been disclosed
- given a copy of the information
- given information on the source of that data.

The patient has the right to rectification if the data is inaccurate. They can apply to court for an order or to the Information Commissioner for an enforcement notice to rectify, block, erase or destroy it. Otherwise, the record can be supplemented by a statement of true facts. A court can order compensation for any harm suffered as a result of inaccuracy.

There is a procedure for access to records and a request must be made in writing to the holder of the records or the data controller, which is usually the NHS Trust, GP or health authority. However, a fee is payable. A response giving the requested information, or stating the grounds for withholding it, must be given within 40 days.

WITHHOLDING INFORMATION

The Data Protection Order[4] modifies the right of access to health records in certain circumstances. This means that the information held in the records may be withheld in certain circumstances; for example:

➤ where the access to the health records is likely to cause serious harm to the physical or mental health or condition of the patient or any other person (which may include a health professional). A data controller who is not a health professional shall not withhold information on these grounds unless he has first consulted the person who appears to be the appropriate health professional about whether this exception applies. The data controller must be prepared to justify any decision to withhold information

➤ where request for access is made by another person on behalf of the data subject, such as a parent for a child

➤ if giving access would reveal the identity of another person, unless that person has given consent to the disclosure or it is reasonable to comply with the access request without that consent. This does not apply if the third party is a health professional who has been involved in the care of the patient, unless serious harm to that health professional's physical or mental health or condition is likely to be caused by giving access.

Certain information can be withheld if it is supplied in a report or other evidence is given to the court by a local authority, health or a social services board, or other person in the course of any proceedings to which various statutes apply (e.g. family proceedings courts) if, under the rules, information can be withheld.

If a patient wishes to see the record, then they should make a request in writing for access. Once the data controller has all the information needed to deal with the request, and is in receipt of the fee, they must consult the appropriate health professional, who is normally the individual who is or was responsible for the clinical care of the patient during the period to which the application refers.

Where there is more than one health professional, the most suitable available health professional should advise on access, otherwise a health professional (with the necessary qualifications and experience) should advise on the matters to which the information requested relates. This will apply to data controllers who are not health professionals.

Where it is agreed that an individual may directly inspect their medical record, access should be supervised by the attendance of a health professional or supervised by a lay administrator. Lay administrators must not comment or advise on the content of the record and, if the applicant raises queries, an appointment with a health professional should be offered.

Where the information is not readily intelligible, an explanation of, for example, abbreviations or medical terminology, must be given.

CHILDREN'S RECORDS

As a general rule, a person with parental responsibility will have the right to apply for access to a child's health record; that is, someone under the age of 18 years.

There are situations in which access to the child's records can be refused. As the child grows older and gains sufficient understanding (known as Fraser Competent), they will be able to make decisions about their own life.

Where a child is considered capable of making decisions about their medical treatment, the consent of the child must be sought before a person with parental responsibility can be given access.

Where, in the view of the appropriate health professional, the child patient is incapable of understanding the nature of the application, the holder of the record is entitled to deny access if it is felt not to be in the patient's best interests to release it.

COPYING LETTERS TO GPs AND PATIENTS

As a result of the government's response to the Kennedy Report (Bristol Enquiry),[5] where letters are written from one health professional to another about a patient, the patient has the right to receive a copy.

The overriding objective is to improve communication with patients and enable them to participate in their care. Patients and carers want information and close involvement in making decisions that affect them. Details of the Kennedy Report and policy are set out below. The policy covers all professionals working in the NHS. All letters concerning NHS patients written about a patient to another health or social care professional should be copied to the patient, if the patient wishes.

Copying letters to patients reinforces the ethic of working in partnership with them and enhances their ability to be more involved in their own healthcare. Patients should have the option of having information about the treatment that is being planned for them. Patients have the right to see their medical records, although in practice much communication between professionals is not available to the patients. Patients often do not know why they are being referred, or what is being said about them. Providing patients with copies of letters between clinicians about individual patients' care will improve the ability of those patients to understand and make choices about their own healthcare and treatment.

Many patients want more information about their own condition and treatment choices, even where there is bad news or a difficult diagnosis or even the suspicion of one. For many, receiving copies of letters helps them remember what they have been told and to share it with family and friends.

In a report of the Working Group on Copying Letters to Patients there is a letter from a patient, which reads:

> 'Thank you for the copy of the letter. It made it seem as if I was more involved with my care. It was easier to talk to the GP about my care, without the problem of trying to remember all that was said at the hospital appointment, which would have been very difficult as I was very nervous at the time. I feel more positive knowing that I am fully informed. It has taken some of the worry of having surgery away by creating a more personal liaison between hospital Consultant and patient.' (From a patient in a pilot project on copying clinicians' letters to patients at Darent Valley Hospital, Dartford and Gravesham NHS Trust.)

For many health professionals, the policy represents a major culture change.

Implementing this policy should be straightforward – a matter of generating an extra copy to a patient whenever a letter about them is written between healthcare professionals.

On closer examination, however, a number of issues arise. They include the exercise of patient choice to receive the letters, data protection and confidentiality, the extent of risk, (for instance in breaching confidentiality and dangers of releasing sensitive information about third parties), particular issues around mental health diagnoses, the rights of carers, parents and children to receive copy letters or other information, provisions for people who lack the mental capacity to make decisions for themselves, the timing of sending or giving the copy letter to a patient and the need to protect patients from clinicians' unconfirmed suspicions – no matter how small – of 'bad news'.

What is important is that the *right* to receive the copy letter should be seen as part of good clinical care, including expectations for good communication between patients and professionals.

Where letters between professionals are routinely copied to patients, potential 'problems' should not be used as an excuse for no action. For instance, concern has been expressed about the possibility of letters being misdirected or seen by someone other than the patient.

As a general rule, where patients agree, all letters written by one health professional to another about a patient should be copied to the patient, including letters written by NHS professionals to outside agencies.

The person writing the letter should be responsible for ensuring a copy is provided to the patient, having confirmed that they wish to receive a copy. This is subject to their consent to do so, which should be noted on their records or in the letter itself. There may be occasions when a patient does not want a letter sent to their home. The patient may decide how they wish to receive it; for example, whether they want to collect it in person or by post.

There are some circumstances where it may be impracticable, unlawful or undesirable to copy letters to patients, including where:
➤ the patient does not want a copy
➤ the letter includes information about or given by a third party
➤ the clinician feels that it may cause potential harm to the patient
➤ the letter contains abnormal results or significant information that has not been discussed with the patient, in which case alternative

arrangements should be made to discuss its contents before providing a copy to the patient, if they so wish.

Copying letters to patients improves the quality of healthcare by:
➤ fostering partnership between patients and health professionals
➤ encouraging patients to be informed and responsible users of health services
➤ increasing the opportunities healthcare providers have to give information to patients
➤ increasing the chances of inaccurate information being corrected.

Professionals have found that copying letters to patients improves communication with patients and carers, increases the likelihood that they will understand and follow advice, and leads to more accurate notes.

Potential benefits of copying letters between professionals to patients

The potential benefits of copying letters between professionals to patients include:
➤ more trust between patients and professionals: increased openness leads to greater trust and openness between professionals and patients
➤ better informed patients: patients and carers have a better understanding of their condition and how they can help themselves
➤ better decisions: patients are more informed and better able to make decisions about treatment options
➤ better compliance: patients who understand the reasons for taking medication or treatment are more likely to follow advice
➤ more accurate records: errors can be spotted and corrected by the patient
➤ better consultations: professionals confirm that patients understand what is said during the consultation; patients are better prepared and less anxious
➤ health promotion: the letters can be used to reinforce advice on self-care and lifestyles.

Patients who do not want a copy

Occasionally patients may not want a letter because:
➤ they feel they already have the information. Where the patient has a

care plan (given as part of the Care Programme Approach, for instance) they may not also want copies of letters
➤ there are problems of privacy at home (e.g. for young people), or there may be domestic violence or information not known to a partner or other members of the household
➤ they do not feel able to accept a diagnosis (e.g. some people with mental health problems).

There are some services (e.g. sexual health clinics) where confidentiality is particularly important and information is not routinely recorded in patients' GP records. The implications of someone else seeing a copy of a letter about treatment by such a service may be serious for the patient, and should be discussed if the patient wants a copy sent by post.

Harm to the patient

Many concerns are raised about copying letters particularly in sensitive areas, such as child protection issues or mental health problems. In some such cases, it may not be appropriate to copy the letter to the patient, although the patient will have the right to request access under the Data Protection Act 1998.

Third party information

Where the letter includes information given by or about a third party (e.g. a neighbour or family member), it is a breach of confidentiality to pass this information onto the patient without the consent of the third party. In such cases, the health professional must comply with the provisions of the Data Protection Act 1998. Sometimes it may be possible to delete that part of the letter that refers to the third party or to include this information as an attachment letter not copied to the patient. If it is not possible to do this, the letter should be withheld and the reasons for this explained to the patient. Patients would have the right to make a 'subject access request' under the provisions of the Data Protection Act 1998. In such cases, it might be helpful to have a standard template letter to explain the situation.

Some third party information may refer to another healthcare professional. Under the Data Protection Act 1998, such information cannot be passed on without the consent of that third party. However, where access to the patient's own information is denied, on such grounds the patient can make a formal access request and information about the health professionals must be disclosed unless there is the likelihood of serious harm to that health professional from disclosure.

There may also be occasions where one healthcare professional wishes to comment on the clinical care provided by another and offer advice on the care of future patients with a particular condition or symptoms. It may not be appropriate for such information to be copied to the patient, but it is important for continuing professional development and clinical governance that such an opportunity for professional development is not lost. The professional concerned should write a separate letter that is not copied to the patient.

However, there could be arguments for copying such information to the patient on the grounds of openness and including the patient in a more open discussion about problems of providing appropriate care.

Patients who cannot give consent

Some people are not able to give consent to receipt of copied letters. Although this type of consent is materially different from that of consent to treatment, as a general rule, practitioners should work within the guidelines on consent produced by professional bodies. The Department of Health gives advice on obtaining consent in different settings and from patients with different needs and competencies.[6]

Mental incapacity

Some people may not have the appropriate mental capacity to make a decision about whether they would like a copy of a letter; for instance, because they have learning difficulties or dementia. It is important, however, not to make 'blanket' assumptions about such incapacity. Whereas it may be judged that a person lacks mental capacity for one purpose, they may have sufficient mental capacity for another.

It should already be recorded on a patient's record if they have someone to act on their behalf or to represent their views – a carer, an advocate or key worker. Advocates can offer independent support where someone, for instance with learning disabilities, needs support in decision-making and wants an alternative to a carer or family member.

Carers

Some people have carers, family members or others who are actively involved in their care. As carers they need information and support from professionals involved in the treatment of the person they care for, and they have a right to an assessment of their own needs through the Carers and Disabled Children Act 2000.[7] Generally, patients want information shared with their carers and, with the patient's consent, copies of letters can be sent to the carer. Copies of letters to carers may be particularly important where medication is changed following discharge from hospital.

However, occasionally, the patient may not want the letter copied or shown to the carer. Both the patient and the carer have the right to expect that information provided to the health service will not be shared with other people without their consent. Unless there is an overriding reason to breach confidentiality, the wishes of the patient must be respected.

Children and young people

Young people aged 16 and 17 are able to make healthcare decisions for themselves,[8] and therefore they should be asked for their consent to receive copies of letters about them. It is up to health professionals to assess the competence of younger children to understand and make a decision (referred to as Fraser competence). It is good practice to offer adolescents consultations on their own, so that they have the opportunity to speak freely and give information that they may be unwilling to talk about in front of their parents. In such cases, young people may prefer copies of letters giving personal information not to be sent to their home.

The issue may arise as to whether a letter should be copied to the young person or their parents. Many existing initiatives in copying letters have been developed in children's services, and the general experience is that there are few difficulties, as long as the issue is discussed with the family. Often adolescents appreciate the letter being sent to them rather than their parents. Where parents are separated, it is important to discuss who should receive copies of letters.

Responsibility for generating and sending the copy

The person who writes the letter should be responsible for ensuring a copy is made and provided to the patient, after confirming:
➤ that the patient wishes to receive a copy
➤ how the patient wishes to receive it
➤ the preferred format (e.g. an exact copy of the letter or a letter explaining what the letter says explaining medical terminology).

The letter itself should make clear what arrangements have been agreed with the patient.

Writing style and standard letters

As a matter of good practice, letters between health professionals, which are copied to patients, should be written clearly. They should not use unnecessarily complex language, and should avoid subjective statements about the patient. They should avoid unnecessary technical terminology and use clear terms without losing their meaning, such as 'kidney' for 'renal' or 'heart attack' for 'myocardial infarction', or explain a technical term in a short additional sentence or phrase. The facts should be set out and unnecessary speculation should be avoided.

They should reinforce and confirm the information given and discussion with the patient in the consultation. Where appropriate, advice on care management (e.g. how to dress a wound), lifestyle changes (e.g. giving up smoking) or treatment options should be included.

Legal scrutiny

If the letter to another health professional is written in such a technical way that the patient cannot understand it, a letter explaining what it means can be sent to the patient. It is important to ensure that there are no inconsistencies between the two letters. Any inconsistencies will expose the health professional to cross-examination should the matter come before the courts.

REFERENCES

1 The Data Protection Act 1998.
2 The Data Protection Act 1984.
3 Access to Health Records Act 1990.
4 The Stationery Office. *The Data Protection (Subject Access Modifications) (Health) Order 2000.* London: The Stationery Office; 2000.
5 Health Service Commissioner. *Learning from Bristol: the Department of Health's response to the report of the public inquiry into children's heart surgery at the Bristol Royal Infirmary 1984–1995.* Available at: www.dh.gov.uk/en/Publicationsandstatistics/Publications/PublicationsPolicyAndGuidance/DH_4002859 (accessed 12 February 2009).
6 The Department of Health. *Good Practice in Consent Implementation Guide: consent to examination and treatment.* Available at: www.dh.gov.uk/en/Publicationsandstatistics/Publications/PublicationsPolicyAndGuidance/DH_4005762 (accessed 12 February 2009).
7 Carers and Disabled Children Act 2000.
8 Family Law Reform Act 1968, S8.

CHAPTER 14

Systems of record keeping

Records must be kept safe and secure. Systems of record keeping are the key to providing good patient care. Health professionals often complain that it takes too long to get the records from the records department or that they cannot locate the documents they need because they have been poorly filed. They may simply be unaware of the existence of certain documents because of poor filing or a delay in filing documents.

In 1999, the Audit Commission reported that hospital patients were being put at risk because their medical histories were kept in a mess and were sometimes lost.[1] The Audit Commission found that out of eight hospitals investigated, half were found to be disorganised.

Medical records staff spent almost two-thirds of their time trying to track down the 36% of files that could not be found in record libraries. About 5% were never located.

In some departments, there was a failure to keep track of files. There was also a failure to protect patient confidentiality. Notes were often found unattended in outpatients' clinics. Sometimes case notes were left on trolleys until the next morning because the medical records office had closed. The report recommended that each hospital should set up a main records library with good security.

The Department of Health, Records Management: NHS code of practice[2] includes guidance on the organisation of the patient record to ensure that a comprehensive system for the completion, use, storage and retrieval of health records is in place.

In a case study, health records at the Weston General Hospital underwent a major revision ahead of the planned introduction of electronic records. They looked at how to reduce the size of the health records and make the actual documentation more concise. They also looked at the way records were filed so that integration with the electronic system could be seamless.

The records were originally set out with four spines divided into:

1 attendances
2 clinical history
3 correspondence
4 results, nursing notes, charts, physiotherapy notes or any other relevant documentation.

They looked at episodic filing: filing by each episode of treatment, rather than by specialty and clinical history. This sets out a complete history of an episode with all the notes relating to it being filed together. Instead of simply listing the dates the patient attended, the record would include an index of all the episodes the patient had ever had. This would make a smooth transition to the new system.

Episodic filing shows continuity of care. When the patient record is accessed there is no need to flip between sections to check, for example, the clinical details or the nursing notes. It is all laid out together in chronological order, so if there are any investigations, all the information is available.

This is likely to improve the quality of patient care. It creates consistency of entries. The records cover demographic details, medical history and what has been agreed already with clinicians, so that the health professionals do not need to ask the same questions time after time. The record is a single document, in which all professionals in the hospital can write, so that they can see what other staff have recorded.

This system of the combined record, where all health professionals record chronologically, is being adopted by many Trusts and is proving to be beneficial. For example, a doctor may request that the patient is seen by an occupational therapist. Where the occupational therapist keeps their own notes, the doctor will be unaware of whether the patient was actually seen, when they were seen and what the outcome was. The doctor may make an assumption that the patient has been seen simply because a referral was made. If the occupational therapist records in the combined record, the doctor will have all of the information and will know whether the patient has been seen and, if they have not, the doctor can chase it up. Communication will undoubtedly be improved and thus patient care will benefit.

SUPPLEMENTARY RECORDS

Wherever possible, concerns should be shared with the patient and the relevant entry in the records should be jointly compiled.

In certain situations it may be appropriate for a health professional to make the entry in a supplementary record to which access by the patient, client or family members is limited or withheld. However, writing in a supplementary record should not become the norm, but happen only in exceptional circumstances. The health professional must be able to justify keeping such a supplementary record. Such records are justified in circumstances where, for example, to write an entry in the patient-held record would put a child or a vulnerable adult at risk.

EXAMPLE OF JUSTIFIABLE SUPPLEMENTARY RECORD

If the health professional were to record details in the patient-held record that a family member poses a risk to a child or vulnerable adult, there is a danger that the next time the health professional attends the home they may be refused entry to the house. This would not only hinder the care of the patient, but could also put the child or vulnerable adult at further risk.

If such entries are recorded in a supplementary record, there must be a system in place for alerting health professionals to the existence of such a record. This will ensure that the information can be accessed readily; it will also enable the health professional to provide the right level of care and to assess the risks.

There may be a risk to health professionals, for example, in community care where there is a history of the patient displaying threatening behaviour towards health professionals in particular. There may be information in the supplementary record that health professionals should only attend the patient's home with a colleague. It is essential that this information be communicated to health professionals. Failure to do so places colleagues at risk. It is too late if they attend the patient's home alone and are injured because the risk was not communicated to them.

ELECTRONIC RECORDS

The rules and responsibilities of record keeping apply equally to both written and electronic records. It is not necessary to keep paper copies of computer-held records. They do not replace the need to maintain a dialogue throughout the healthcare team. Safeguards for computer-held records must be in compliance with the Computer Misuse Act 1990.[3]

The use of information technology to record the planning, assessment and delivery of care is increasing. A computer-held record system has enormous potential benefits for patients. Electronic records tend to be easier to read and less bulky, reduce the need for duplication and can increase communication between members of the inter-professional healthcare team. It allows health professionals, wherever they may be, to have instant, accurate access to patients' health history, including allergies, current medication, pre-existing conditions, recent treatment and appointments. They will link hospitals, GP surgeries and other agencies.

We have seen the difficulties caused by fragmented documentation in the case study in Chapter 4. Electronic records may be the solution to this, with the promise by the government of a system of integrated care records and national standards.[4]

In some areas of healthcare the use of electronic records is increasingly the norm. They can be of enormous assistance to health professionals.

The Department of Health published 'Clear Rules Set Out for Patients' Electronic Records',[5] which sets out a guarantee and makes 12 commitments to patients about their records, including the following pledges:

➤ access to records by NHS staff will be strictly limited to those having a 'need to know' to provide effective treatment to a patient

➤ in due course, patients will be able to block off parts of their record to stop its being shared with anyone in the NHS, except in an emergency

➤ individuals will be able to stop their information being seen by anyone outside the organisation that created it – although doing so may have an impact on the quality of care they receive.

Potentially, electronic records have the advantage over manual records of making important information faster and easier to access; they also avoid the problem of illegibility and should reduce spelling errors. However, the principles of good record keeping still apply to the content, clarity and accuracy of the information.

Computer-held records are being implemented incrementally. In some areas, computer-held records run alongside the written records. In many departments, the written record is then typed up onto the computer.

In some circumstances someone other than the health professional providing the care and writing the manual record enters the information into the computer record. This may be an administrator or another health professional who did not provide the care. They take the information from the manual record, but this can be a problem because they do not have first-hand knowledge of what happened, and this leaves room for error. They may misinterpret the information or transpose it inaccurately. Where there are gaps in the detail they may simply fill in those gaps by making assumptions.

Sometimes the computer system requires all fields to be completed, resulting in the temptation to complete them by making assumptions.

EXAMPLE OF AN ASSUMPTION WHEN INPUTTING COMPUTER RECORDS

In a set of records from a maternity department, one of the questions on the system asks whether syntocinon has been administered to the patient. This drug is sometimes used for inducing labour, but may also be used to combat excessive uterine bleeding postpartum. The records noted that the patient's labour had been induced, although it did not record how. The person inputting the details into the electronic records made an assumption that because labour had been induced, the patient must have been administered syntocinon for this purpose. This was an incorrect assumption.

Another time for caution is where there is a tick box for stating, for example, which medication has been prescribed or administered. If offered a range of options it is very easy to tick box A instead of box B, compared to the manual record where it is less likely that a health professional will erroneously write 'paracetamol' instead of 'syntocinon'.

Incompatibility

Other difficulties currently faced by health professionals are that current systems used by various Trusts, GPs and other agencies are incompatible and information cannot be accessed or transferred between them.

Confidentiality

Another issue that health professionals need to be aware of is that there must be very strict controls on who has access to patients' records, to ensure that health information is kept confidential.

Accountability

When a health professional makes an entry in the record, either manual or electronic, they will be accountable for the entry. The health professional must ensure that all entries are clearly identifiable. Therefore, health professionals should not leave their computer logged on in their name, which could allow others to access the system. Likewise, other health professionals or administrative staff should not use someone else's log-in details to access the system.

Amending electronic records

The system should be set up in such a way that health professionals cannot amend entries retrospectively. They should be dealt with in the same way as a manual record. If something has been left out of an entry and is entered later, the health professional should explain why it has been done retrospectively.

In the unlikely event that the records are viewed as being suspicious, an audit trail is carried out. The system records when the entries were made and amended and it can track those changes. This was, of course, the compelling evidence used in the Shipman trial, where the computer system showed that Shipman had made retrospective entries to cover his tracks.[6]

Although the electronic records have their advantages there are still some difficulties surrounding the implementation of the electronic systems. There has been much controversy regarding the cost and delays of implementation. Different Trusts use different systems and these systems are not compatible with each other so that electronic records cannot be transferred with the patient to a new Trust. Similarly, GP practices do not use a unified system. The government is working towards integrated care records to improve patient care.[7-9]

REFERENCES

1 The Audit Commission. *The Audit Commission Report: setting the record straight.* Available at: www.audit-commission.gov.uk/reports/ (accessed 12 February 2009).
2 The Department of Health. *Records Management: NHS Code of Practice.* Dated 05/04/06. Available at: www.dh.gov.uk
3 Computer Misuse Act 1990.
4 Royal College of Nursing. *Computerised patient records – what can they offer?* 29 March 2007. Available at: www.rcn.org.uk/newsevents/congress/2008/2007_agenda_items/18_computerised_patient_records (accessed 4 June 2007).
5 The Department of Health. *Clear Rules Set Out for Patients' Electronic Records.* 23 May 2005. Available at: www.dh.gov.uk/en/Publicationsandstatistics/pressrelease/DH_4111988 (acessed 23 February 2009).
6 Dame Janet Smith. *The Fourth Report: the regulation of controlled drugs in the community.* July 2004. Available at: www.the-shipman-inquiry.org.uk/fourthreport.asp (accessed 12 February 2009).
7 Department of Health. *Integrated Mental Health Electronic Record (IMHER).* January 2001. Available at: www.dh.gov.uk/en/Publicationsandstatistics/Publications/PublicationsPolicyAndGuidance/DH_4126633 (accessed 12 February 2009).
8 Department of Health. *Electronic Social Care Record.* 23 November 2007. Available at: www.dh.gov.uk/en/Managingyourorganisation/Informationpolicy/Informationforsocialcare/DH_4073714 (accessed 23 February 2009).
9 Department of Health. *The Government Response to the Health Committee Report on the Electronic Patient Record.* November 2007. Available at: www.dh.gov.uk/en/Publicationsandstatistics/Publications/PublicationsPolicyAndGuidance/DH_080238 (accessed 12 February 2009).

CHAPTER 15

Further considerations

INFECTION CONTROL AND THE RECORDS

Infection control has become a major concern to patients and health professionals. All health professionals should be familiar with their employer's policies and guidelines about infection control and ensure that they are followed.

It is important that there is evidence in the records that these policies and procedures have been adhered to. The records should clearly note if the patient is cohorted; that is, whether the patient is being kept separate or grouped with other same sufferers to avoid the spread of infection. It is also important to ensure that other documentation and any notifications are adhered to and recorded. For example, cases of *Clostridium difficile* (*C. diff*) should be recorded in the relevant registers, and staff, such as bed managers, should be notified. Such notifications should also be recorded in the patient's notes.

MENTAL HEALTH RECORDS

Health professionals working with patients who are subject to mental health legislation must ensure that they have a thorough working knowledge of the statutory powers as they apply to their area of practice. When making entries in records for these patients, they must comply as appropriate with the guidance given by the Mental Health Act Commission for England and

Wales,[1] the Mental Welfare Commission for Scotland[2] or the Mental Health Commission for Northern Ireland.[3]

Where records relate to the detention and treatment of mentally disordered patients, statutory provisions apply to what must be recorded, in what circumstances and how corrections can be made. If there is a failure to comply with the statutory provisions relating to detention, the patient would not be lawfully detained and could seek his or her release. The Mental Health Act 1983[4] and regulations made under this Act seek to ensure that records of the detention of mentally disordered patients are kept to a high standard.

The Mental Health Act 1983 and statutory instruments make it compulsory to use specified documentation for the detention and compulsory treatment of patients. Forms have been drawn up by the Department of Health and they are used for a specific purpose. It is important to stress that these documents cannot be amended, subject to strict exceptions. They may be rectified only in limited circumstances as set out under Section 15 of the Mental Health Act 1983.[5] More detail can be found on page 99, 'Amending the records'.

Where a patient is admitted voluntarily to a psychiatric hospital, there are no statutory provisions, but the general principles of good practice in record keeping apply.

Records dealing with mental health issues can be more difficult to write due to the less tangible nature of the content. Often the issues involve emotion rather than more physical presentations, such as blood pressure or temperature. This can be particularly difficult when writing process notes, which include feelings, as opposed to clinical notes. Where entries include how the health professional is feeling, this must be clearly distinguished from the feelings of the patient.

It is important to keep information factual, and not to record, for example, 'the patient is depressed' unless you are qualified to do so, as this is a clinical diagnosis. If the patient says they are depressed, this should be recorded as a fact: 'the patient said she felt depressed'.

When considering how much to write, health professionals should have particular regard to the of detail deemed important to the health professional. They may wish to record and retain a transcript of the whole consultation in full.

Where risk to the patient is an issue (e.g. self-harm, abuse of a child or older person or risk of violence to the public at large), seemingly minor details assume greater significance. It is important in these circumstances to make a more detailed record.

Remember the same good practice record keeping guide applies to mental health records, so dates and timings and so on must be recorded.

EXAMPLE OF THE NECESSITY OF RECORDING DATES AND TIMES

If the health professional sees a patient who later commits suicide, the timings of the entries will be crucial in determining how long after the patient was seen by the health professional the patient took their own life.

MIDWIFERY RECORDS

As with other records, the primary purpose of midwifery records is to document the treatment, care and support of the mother and baby. However, there is a high incidence of complaints and legal disputes in relation to maternity care. Accordingly, midwives are highly likely to have to give an explanation in response to a complaint, and evidence in court. The midwife's records will be required and will be relied upon as evidence.

If a child is injured or dies as a result of negligent treatment at birth, a claim for compensation may be brought. It can take many years for a claim to come to court and the midwife will therefore have to give evidence about an incident that occurred many years previously. The midwife may even have retired from practice.

Therefore, information about care provided must be clearly and accurately noted in these records. The same good practice guide applies to these records. In addition, Rule 9 of the *Midwives Rules*',[6] which came into force on 1 August 2004, emphasises that the records relating to the care of the women and babies are an essential aspect of practice to aid communication between the health professional, the women and others who are providing care. They demonstrate the standard of care provided.

There is other documentation specific to midwives; for example, cardio-tachograph (CTG) records. These should be retained along with any other records. Where significant events occur these can be recorded on the graph itself. The advantage of this is that the graph is timed so the midwife does not need to write in the time again. However, the CTG clock must be checked to ensure that it is the correct time (*see* the section on time at page 85). In addition, some equipment allows the machine itself to record significant events if the appropriate buttons are pressed.

Notwithstanding the high incidence of litigation, midwifery records should not be written defensively with the court in mind. They should be written for the benefit of treating, caring and supporting the mother and baby.

SOCIAL CARE RECORDS

Over the last 25 years, inadequate case records have often been cited as a factor in cases with tragic outcomes. A report from of the Department of Health highlighted the need to improve case recording in social services departments (SSDs).[7] Inspections of case records in seven departments showed that generally insufficient management attention had been paid to recording. The report identified the shortcomings and provided a benchmark for best practice, including aspects of sharing and access, elements of an effective record, information technology, management and training and audit tools in the form of checklists focusing on policy and practice.

Good case recording is an important part of the accountability of staff working in SSDs to those who use their services. It helps to focus the work of staff and it supports effective partnerships with service users and carers. It ensures there is a documented account of a department's involvement with individual service users, families and carers. It assists continuity when workers are unavailable or there are staff changes, and provides an essential tool for managers to monitor work.

The purpose of case records is to be used by care managers and care workers as an effective tool for communicating. They are a major source of evidence for investigations and formal inquiries and are used by other professionals like health, police, education or other contributors to provide proper safeguards.

The case record should ensure that staff can account for work done. It is a source of wider information that will be relied upon by others for making policy and may be used as an analytical and supervisory tool.

Case records are essential for managers to monitor the work done with users, and for the recording of decisions taken. They can use the record to ensure continuity when a worker changes or is unavailable.

Case files and case records

The differences between case files and case records need to be made clear.

The case file is the folder that contains all the information about an individual or a family that has been referred to an SSD and accepted as a 'case' for allocation and further action. The information may comprise letters, financial statements and reports from other agencies, legal documents and a variety of other items. It helps to organise different categories of information into different sections in the file so that each piece of information is easily accessible. Computer records may be copied on to the main file or held on computer.

The case record is the written account of the SSD's work with an individual or family, which details the individual contacts with the service user, the work to be done and its objectives, the procedure to be followed, the assessment of need, the case plan, the timing, process and outcomes of reviews.

Detail

The same regard to detail must be given as in any other care record (as discussed in previous Chapters 5, 6, 7, 8, 9 and 10). Detail in social records is paramount. Health and social care professionals, the courts and others will be making significant decisions affecting the lives of children, vulnerable adults and others based upon the records.

It is important that they reflect accurately and factually without bias or subjectivity. Research shows that often a good standard of care is delivered yet the records do not reflect it. The records should reflect the standard of care that was actually provided.

The quality of case records may materially affect the ability of the local authority to present evidence properly in matters that come before the courts, or to present an accurate account of its actions in other judicial proceedings or inquiries or for insurance claims against the local authority. This is crucial, for example, when matters of child protection are being contemplated. It is important for local authorities to be confident that recording practice conforms to local and national policies, and reflects the best interests of the community they serve.[8]

REFERENCES

1 www.mhac.org.uk
2 www.mwcscot.org.uk
3 www.mhcni.org
4 The Mental Health Act 1983.
5 The Mental Health Act 1983, S15.
6 The Nursing and Midwifery Council. *Midwives' Rules and Standards*. Available at: www.nmc-uk.org/aFrameDisplay.aspx?DocumentID=169 (accessed 10 February 2009).
7 Department of Health. *Recording with Care: inspection of case recording in social services departments report*. January 1999. Available at: www.dh.gov.uk/en/Publicationsandstatistics/Publications/PublicationsPolicyAndGuidance/DH_4010129 (accessed 12 February 2009).
8 Ibid.

CHAPTER 16

Who owns the health records?

Where an organisation employs professional staff who make records, the organisation is the legal owner of those records. Thus, an NHS Trust will own the health records made by those working for them. This does not mean, however, that anyone in the organisation has an automatic right of access to the records or the information contained within them.

Health professionals have a duty to protect the confidentiality of the patient or client record. This is particularly important when there are potential areas of conflict, such as occupational health records, where the record itself belongs to the organisation, but the information contained in the record is confidential and should only be released, even to someone within the organisation, with the consent of the patient or client.

PATIENT-HELD RECORDS

Patients and clients increasingly own their healthcare records, particularly in community care, and this should be encouraged as far as it is appropriate and as long as they are happy to do so. This enables the patient to be more closely involved in their own care and enables the health professional to share with them the information that is considered relevant to the patient's assessment and care. Patients should be informed of the purpose and importance of the record and their responsibility for keeping it safe. These same principles apply equally to parent-held records.

SUPPLEMENTARY RECORDS

Where the health professional feels that particular concerns or anxieties require them to keep supplementary records to which access by the patient, client or family members is limited or withheld, these records are owned by the organisation or owned by the health professional, if that person is self-employed.

STORAGE OF HEALTH RECORDS

The requirement for keeping records for a specified period of time is dependent upon a number of pieces of legislation including, amongst others, the Limitation Act 1980[1] and the Congenital Disabilities (Civil Liability) Act 1976.[2] Retention of records is also governed by health services policy statements issued by government health departments.

It is a requirement that health providers have a policy in place for retention and storage of health records. It is the practice of most healthcare providers to keep the records for periods that vary between 6 years (after the last entry) and 25 years. Trust policies usually require health professionals to retain records for at least 8 years and, in the case of a child, until the child's 21st birthday at least. Mental health records should be retained for longer periods.

Where the health professional is self-employed, they should also ensure that no record made relating to the care of a patient or client is destroyed within a period of 8 years after the last entry or 21 years for children's records.

Records are kept for these periods of time for reasons of patient care, but also in case they are required as evidence. The Limitation Act 1980 sets out the time frames for potential claimants to bring a civil action and judges have the discretion to waive the limitation period.

As set out in Chapter 18 entitled 'Health records used as evidence', if a civil claim were to be brought by a patient, as a civil action is a dispute between two parties, the judge will determine the case on the balance of probabilities. In other words, who has the best evidence and whose evidence does the judge prefer? The claimant who, on oath, genuinely remembers and believes everything or the health professional who remembers little or nothing?

If there is a contradiction between what is remembered and what was recorded in the contemporaneously written record, it is usually the records that are preferred over the claimant's oral testimony. It is not putting it too strongly to say that whether a case is won or lost will depend on the quality and detail of the record. It is therefore vital that the records are sufficiently detailed to enable the health professional, when giving evidence, to reconstruct precisely what happened from those notes. The court says that if it is not recorded, then it didn't happen.

It follows that the destruction of records exposes the health professional to an adverse finding because, in the absence of the records, there will be no evidence to show the standard of care provided. Regard should therefore be given to the Limitation Act 1980[1] in determining the length of time that records should be stored.

The point relates to the time frame for the storage of documentation. The Limitation Act 1980 sets out the time frames for aggrieved persons to bring an action. There is judicial discretion to disapply any limitation under Section 33 of the Limitation Act 1980.[3]

The Act lays down the maximum period in which a person who has suffered a personal injury may bring a claim; that is, up to three years from the date on which the incident occurred or three years from the date of knowledge that the incident caused the injury (if later).

The date of knowledge can sometimes be difficult to determine.

EXAMPLE OF DATE OF KNOWLEDGE

A patient undergoes surgery in January 1995. Following the surgery, the patient has a history of stomach pain. In February 2005 the patient undergoes further surgery during which the surgeon finds an instrument that had been left behind in the 1995 operation. It is this retained instrument that has been the cause of the ongoing pain.

Although the incident (the instrument being retained) occurred in 1995, the patient's date of knowledge will be February 2005 when the retained instrument was discovered and the patient then knew that it was this that had caused the ongoing pain. The patient has three years from the February 2005 date (i.e. until February 2008) to commence court proceedings.

Deceased

If the person injured dies before the expiration of the three-year period then the limitation date is three years from the date of death or three years from the date of knowledge of the personal representatives for the estate, whichever is later. For example, the personal representatives dealing with the probate may learn from an inquest that the death was caused by a medical error. The three-year date of knowledge will run from the date of the inquest.

Section 33

Section 33 of the Limitation Act 1980[4] gives the court discretion to disapply the time limit for bringing a claim in certain circumstances. This discretion is often used where the patient suffers from, for example, a mental disability.

Minor

A person under the age of 18 years is a minor and the Limitation Act 1980 allows a minor to bring a claim within three years from the date of the incident or three years from the age of attaining majority, whichever is later.

For example, if a child suffers an injury at the age of 8 years they have until the age of 21 to bring a claim. It is usual for a child's records to be stored for up to 25 years.

Mental health records

Storage of documents relating to the detention of patients is set out under the provisions of Section 17 of the National Health Service Act 1977[5] where the Secretary of State has directed that health authorities (extended to Trusts by a direction HC (91) (29)[6] must keep all records required to be made under the 1983 Mental Health Regulations[7] for not less than five years, commencing on the date on which the person to whom they relate ceases to be a hospital patient.

Midwifery records

The NMC states that midwifery/maternity records are required to be retained for a period of 25 years. This is in accordance with the Congenital Disabilities (Civil Liability) Act 1976[8] and applies to England, Wales and Northern Ireland. Scotland has made similar provisions through the Scottish Law Commission. This Act enables a child who is born alive to sue any person, except the mother, who has caused him/her to be born disabled as a result of an act of negligence. (There is one exception to the rule against a child suing their mother; this is where they have been damaged in utero in a car accident as a result of the mother driver not wearing her seat belt).

The Department of Health[9] also recommends that, as a minimum, all obstetric and midwifery records, including those episodes of maternity care that end in stillbirth or where a child later dies, should be kept for 25 years. However, if there is any sign that the child is brain damaged or suffers from a mental disability, those records should be retained until after the death of that person.

All essential maternity records should be retained for professional use and for any investigation under the Congenital and Disabilities (Civil Liabilities) Act 1976.[10] Local policy must specify the particular records to be retained. These will include booking data and pre-pregnancy records, antenatal visits and examinations, antenatal in-patient records, clinical test results including ultrasound scans, CTG, alpha feto protein and chorionic villus sampling, blood test reports, all intrapartum records, prescription records, and postnatal records relating to mother and baby. Other documents to be retained include work diaries if they contain clinical information.

Local policy should also set out details about other records, such as diaries and duty rotas, the transfer and storage of records, including the community midwife's records, and also the return of the records held by the mother during her pregnancy.

The Department of Health[11] suggests minimum periods for the retention of records, some of which are set out in Table 16.1 below.

TABLE 16.1 Minimum periods for record retention

Records	Retention period
General	Eight years after conclusion of treatment
Oncology	Eight years after the conclusion of treatment where only surgery is involved
	Permanent retention electronically where treatment involves chemotherapy and radiotherapy
Abortion certificates A and B	Three years
Children and young people	Until a child's 25th birthday or until the young person's 26th birthday if the person was 17 years of age at the conclusion of the treatment or eight years after the patient's death if it occurred before their 18th birthday
Mentally disordered person (as defined under the Mental Health Act)	20 years after no further treatment is considered necessary
	Eight years after the patient's death if the patient died whilst receiving treatment
Donor records	11 years after the donation
Clinical trials	15 years after conclusion of the treatment

This is not an exhaustive list and further details can be obtained from the Department of Health.[12]

Records to be retained include all health records, x-rays, scans and other records such as diaries, rotas and signature sheets, amongst others.

Health professionals and Trusts must consider how confidentiality will be maintained with regard to the retention and destruction of records.

Records and exhibits should be retained even after the conclusion of legal proceedings, as they may be needed in any appeal process.

REFERENCES

1 Limitation Act 1980.
2 Congenital Disabilities (Civil Liability) Act 1976.
3 Limitation Act 1980, S33.
4 Ibid.
5 National Health Service Act 1977, S17.
6 National Health Service Act 1977 direction HC (91) (29).
7 Mental Health Regulations 1983.
8 Congenital Disabilities op. cit.
9 Department of Health. *For the Record: managing records in NHS Trusts and health authorities.* 19 March 1999. Available at: www.dh.gov.uk/en/Publicationsandstatistics/ Lettersandcirculars/Healthservicecirculars/DH_4003513 (accessed 23 February 2009).
10 Congenital Disabilities op. cit.
11 Department of Health op. cit.
12 Ibid.

CHAPTER 17

Health records used to prepare witness statements and reports

Health professionals may be required to write a witness statement or a report for many reasons; for example:

➤ for a civil court relating to a claim for compensation
➤ for a criminal court relating to child protection issues
➤ for an employment tribunal
➤ for an inquest
➤ for an internal report following an incident
➤ where there has been a complaint by a patient.

There are different types of statements and reports. They serve different purposes and are different in their content and structure. The health professional needs to be aware of the differences before compiling them.

A STATEMENT, REPORT OR EXPERT REPORT?

The difference between the three documents are:

➤ **a witness statement** of fact assists the court by giving a factual account of events
➤ **a report** assists the court by giving facts and opinion where a health professional has been involved in the care or support of the patient
➤ **an expert report** is prepared by a specialist in a particular field who is asked by the court to give an independent opinion on the facts of a case and who is not otherwise involved in the case.

If there is a complaint by a patient or you are involved in legal proceedings it begins with a request for a witness statement. In order to construct a witness statement you need good records. It is those records that will then be turned into the witness statement of fact.

The purpose of a statement is to allow you to assist the court by presenting the facts as they are known to you. Amongst other things, the court will want to know the detail. The court will not be interested in the generality of matters; it will not be interested in what you usually do, what you would have done or could have done; it will want to know the detail of what actually happened in this case.

Your statement must deal with the issues and set out the facts and you must support those facts. If you say 'the patient was in pain', the question is 'how do you know this?' Your statement should say so and be supported by the evidence. For example, the statement ought to say, 'In a telephone call on 3 March 2004 at 15.05 hours the patient told me that he was in pain'.

The records will be needed to reconstruct the detail. As time passes, memory fades and detail fades. Legal cases can sometimes take many years to come to trial so the records will be an essential tool to help you in preparing the statement.

An important matter often not appreciated by the health professional is that when a request for a statement is received, the health professional may assume that the statement is just a note to their boss or the complaints department. In practice, if the matter proceeds to a hearing, the statement is re-written in a much more formal way in line with the Civil Procedure Rules (CPR).[1] It is often not appreciated that the first statement may be disclosed to the court. The court will then look for discrepancies between the original statement and the formal one.

Do not attempt to write the statement without the benefit of the records. Always obtain them and refer to them. This will ensure accuracy of the statement. The opposition lawyers will go through your statement with a fine-tooth comb and look for discrepancies between the records and your statement.

You will recall the case I referred to earlier in Chapter 4, with the discrepancies between the statement and the records, and the difficulties that such discrepancies posed for the Trust and the individuals.

There is a skill in preparing statements, but the details of content and style are not covered within the ambit of this book.

REFERENCE

1   www.justice.gov.uk/civil/procrules_fin/

CHAPTER 18

Health records used as evidence

WILL YOUR RECORDS STAND UP TO LEGAL SCRUTINY?

Health records may be used in a variety of different ways, unforeseen by the writer when the entry was made. Whilst the primary purpose of the records is to facilitate the treatment, care and support of the patient, considerable reliance will be placed upon the records at any court hearing. Any weakness in the records will hinder the health professional when it comes to giving evidence in the witness box. The health professional will be vulnerable under cross-examination especially if there are discrepancies between the documents, errors, or omissions or delays between events occurring and the records of these being documented.

As time passes memories fade and the court will want to know how, after the passage of time, you can recall the information.

When records are accurate they will probably never come to the attention of and be scrutinised by a lawyer. When you are busy the notes reflect this. This is what the lawyers will be looking for; they will be looking at the poor notes.

Records which are unconnected with the patient may be looked at; for example, in the case of Deacon v McVicar[1] there was a dispute with regard to the priority of a patient, and the court ordered the disclosure of records of other patients on the same ward in order to assess whether or not other patients were making demands on medical and nursing time at a particular point.

Health professionals may become involved in the court process in many ways. In all of the court forums, the health records will usually be relied on as evidence. Of course, the notes are clearly a tool to provide patient care and that is their primary purpose. They also have an evidential role. Long after the health professional has finished with the records they may be required to respond to a complaint or for an enquiry for the purpose of litigation.

I am sure most health professionals would agree that when something goes awry with patient care, the patient will remember everything in great detail – who said what to whom, who was there at the time, what they were wearing, and so on. This is unsurprising because for the patient it is an unusual experience – a one-off; it was intensely personal for them and it may have impacted greatly on their life.

The problem for the health professional is that they will have seen a great number of patients and it is doubtful whether they will remember particular events. This is not surprising as many months or years may have passed before the complaints or issues arise. The difficulty for the health professional is that, for the patient, it will have been important and they will have relived and retold the event in great detail and all of the circumstances will be firmly fixed in their memory. When giving evidence the patient will be very compelling, whereas for the health professional, unless there was something very unusual or untoward about the matter that makes it stick in the memory, the detail will have been forgotten or at best will have merged into the background of a busy caseload.

Where a case comes before the civil court, such as a claim for compensation, the court has to determine the outcome. In such cases, it is a dispute between two parties where one party has to win and the other party has to lose. A judge will determine the case on the balance of probabilities. The judge will decide which person has the best evidence and who should be believed.

When a court is faced with a claimant who, on oath, remembers everything, against a health professional who remembers little or nothing at all, the judge has little option but to accept the claimant's version.

While there is little doubt that the patient genuinely believes the accuracy of his recollection, with the passage of time and in the reliving and retelling of the events, the version will have been rationalised and edited, so that whilst the patient believes the version they are recounting to be wholly accurate, it may in fact be wholly inaccurate. The memory is fallible; there is nothing sinister in this. It is simply the way the memory works.

In the absence of any evidence to contradict what the patient said, their version of events will prevail. The only way the presumption that the claimant is right can be overcome is with the records. If there is a contradiction between what is remembered and what was contemporaneously recorded, it is likely that the records will be preferred. Whether a case is won or lost will depend on the quality and detail of the record.

It is important that there is sufficient detail in the records to enable the health professional, when giving evidence, to reconstruct precisely what happened.

As I have said many times in this book, the court's view is, 'if it's not in the notes, then it didn't happen, was not done or was not said'.

UNTRUE OR FALSE ENTRIES

Records used in evidence will be taken at face value and considered true, as they have been written by professionals. The court could place considerable reliance upon their accuracy. However, erroneous entries may in fact have been written accidentally or even deliberately.

In practice, the judge would decide, in light of the evidence given by the witnesses, the weight that will be placed upon the accuracy and comprehensiveness of the records. If the records have deliberately been falsified then this may constitute fraud or dishonesty. The record writer would be accountable and this could be punishable by disciplinary action, fitness to practise proceedings or even perjury in court.

CASE STUDY

A casualty nurse, who had told the parents of a sick baby that he probably had a sniffle and they should take him to the family doctor, altered the notes when the baby died an hour later.[2]

She changed the words 'extremely pale' to 'quite pale' and added a pulse reading even though she had not taken his pulse.

Even though an independent inquiry found that her actions probably had no bearing on the child's outcome, she faced internal disciplinary proceedings at which she was dismissed. Such circumstances could also lead to professional conduct proceedings with the possibility of being struck from the register of the NMC.

MISSING RECORDS

If the records are not available because they are missing or the records were never completed, the courts will have to rely on the best alternative evidence. There may be other records to fill in the gaps, such as ambulance records, which may, for example, have the times of admissions recorded where the admission times are missing from the other records.

Where a party to the case deliberately destroys or loses the records then an adverse inference may be made by the court.

WHAT IS THE COURT LOOKING FOR?

If there is a contradiction between what is remembered and what was recorded in the contemporaneously written records, it is usually the records that are preferred over the claimant's oral testimony. It is not stating it too strongly to say that the quality and detail of the record can determine whether a case is won or lost. It is therefore important that there is sufficient information in the notes to enable the health professional, when giving evidence, to reconstruct from those notes precisely what happened.

In the case of Wisniewski v Central Manchester Health Authority 1998,[3] the court considered the effect of a party failing to bring evidence in support of its case. The court said:

'(1) In certain circumstances a court may be entitled to draw adverse inferences from the absence or silence of a witness who might be expected to have material evidence to give on an issue in an action.

(2) If a court is willing to draw such inferences they may go to strengthen the evidence adduced on that issue by the other party or to weaken the evidence, if any, adduced by the party who might reasonably have been expected to call the witness.

(3) There must, however, have been some evidence, however weak, adduced by the former on the matter in question before the court is entitled to draw the desired inference: in other words, there must be a case to answer on that issue.

(4) If the reason for the witness's absence or silence satisfies the court then no such adverse inference may be drawn. If, on the other hand, there is some

credible explanation given, even if it is not wholly satisfactory, the potentially detrimental effect of his/her absence or silence may be reduced or nullified.'

Put simply, and as I've mentioned a number of times, the court's view is that if it is not recorded, then it did not happen, was not said or was not done.

The court will also look for discrepancies between the different witness statements that have been prepared by the health professional. Remember, anything you write has the potential to become a legal document. The court will look for discrepancies between the various documents.

LACK OF PROFESSIONALISM

There is another aspect of record keeping which must be borne in mind. Long before witnesses are seen or statements are exchanged, the notes will have been read by the lawyers and a view will have been formed about the professionalism or otherwise of the writer. If the notes are clearly unprofessional, it is a very short step to suggest that the same lack of professionalism extended to the care and treatment of the patient.

On one occasion notes were produced for the court where the last entry about the patient read, 'she is mad' (*see* Figure 18.1) and was accompanied by a cartoon drawing. Little had the writer thought that one day the judge and lawyers would be scrutinising this note.

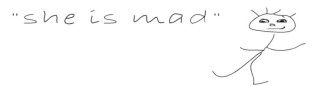

FIGURE 18.1 'She is mad'

Everything that is written in the course of your work has the potential status of a legal document and may one day be scrutinised by the court. If the records are maintained in such an unprofessional way, it will be difficult, if not impossible, to retain professional credibility.

REFERENCES
1 Deacon v McVicar 1984 unreported QBD.
2 Wilkinson P. Notes on dead baby altered by nurse. *The Times*. 7 November 1995.
3 Wisniewski v Central Manchester Health Authority [1998] Lloyds Rep Med 223.

CHAPTER 19

Defensive writing

Health records are written for the purpose of treating, supporting and caring for the patient. They are the tool of communication between professionals, patients and carers. However, it has been identified that too often notes seem to be written with medico-legal rather than communication purposes in mind. Defensive record keeping can easily become poor record keeping. This renders decision making opaque and difficult to defend against challenge.[1]

Health professionals should not be tempted to write the records defensively or to write the notes with litigation in mind. There is a danger that the records will become stylised, verbose or convey different messages from those intended. Remember, the purpose of the records is to facilitate the care, treatment and support of the patient. If they are written defensively there is a danger we move away from their real purpose. This may then result in a breakdown in communication.

An example of what can happen when records are written with lawyers in mind was contained in a report following an incident, which read, *'When the gunmen burst into the department, all the patients evacuated themselves'*. Maybe they did, but it is unlikely that is what the writer intended to convey!

The healthcare professional delivering day-to-day care must make decisions. Although each decision is under review and there is an increasing tendency in society to litigate, they should keep this fear of law in perspective, and not be overly concerned about litigation.

The danger is that if healthcare professionals become too preoccupied with the law and legal issues, they become 'mini lawyers' and put legal considerations before their normal professional duties. Healthcare professionals should never try to become 'mini lawyers'. It is paramount that they act in their own professional role. If the records are written professionally for the purpose of treating, caring and supporting the patient, then the records will be more than adequate for use in court.

REFERENCE
1 Mandelstam M. *An A-Z of Community Care Law.* London: Jessica Kingsley; 1998. p. 163.

CHAPTER 20

Assessment criteria for health records

This is a guide you may find useful and you may wish to adapt it to suit your own needs.

Has the following been recorded:	Yes/No
• Date • Time • Retrospective entry (distinguish time patient seen and time entry written)	
Each entry authenticated: • Signed • Name printed • Designation • Can easily be identified	
• Written as soon as possible after an event has occurred • Chronological order (explanation if written retrospectively)	
• Factual • Consistent • Accurate	
• Current information on the care and condition of the patient or client • Identify problems • Action taken to rectify them • People present (consider: nurse, chaperone, interpreter, multidisciplinary, family)	

(*continued*)

Has the following been recorded:	Yes/No
Clear evidence of: • Care planned • Rationale • Decisions made • Information shared • Follow up	
• Written clearly and in such a manner that the text cannot be erased	
Alterations or additions are: • Dated • Timed • Signed • In such a way that the original entry can still be read clearly	
• No abbreviations • No jargon • No meaningless phrases • No irrelevant speculation • No bias, speculation or offensive subjective statements	
• Legible • Grammatically correct • Spelling correct	
• Written in black ink preferably • Readable on any photocopies	
• Written in terms that the patient or client can understand	
• Clear reference to related documentation • Clear reference to related products or equipment	
Other comments	

Glossary

Accountability	Someone who is accountable is completely responsible for what they do and must be able to give a satisfactory reason for it.
Act of Parliament	A document that sets out legal rules.
Assault and battery	Assault is an intentional or reckless act that causes someone to expect to be subjected to immediate physical harm. Battery is an intentional or negligent application of physical force.
Balance of probability	Establishing the facts to the satisfaction of the court. The standard of proof in civil proceedings is on the balance of probabilities.
Breach of duty	An act of breaking a law. Where there is a duty of care and that duty has not been met. Negligence is also referred to as a breach of the duty of care.
Beyond reasonable doubt	Establishing the facts to the satisfaction of the court. The standard of proof in criminal proceedings is beyond reasonable doubt.
Cauda equina	The nerves at the base of the spine. Cauda equina syndrome is caused by the compression of lumbosacral nerve roots and results in neuromuscular, urinary and bowel symptoms. It is a medical emergency and immediate referral for investigation and treatment is required to prevent permanent neurological damage.

CHI	Commission for Health Improvement.
Chorionic villus sampling	Chorionic villus sampling (CVS) is an invasive diagnostic test for pregnant women. It involves taking a small sample of the placenta and testing it for genetic disorders.
Civil law	The legal system that relates to personal matters, such as marriage and property, rather than criminal matters.
Claimant	A person who brings a claim – sues for something which they believe they have a right to.
Clinical management plan (CMP)	Is a document that must be used before supplementary prescribing can take place. It can be hand written or electronic.
Clostridium difficile	(*C. diff*) is an infection caused by bacteria. Symptoms include diarrhoea and other more serious conditions that affect the gut. The infection often occurs after someone has taken antibiotics to treat another illness.
Cohorted	Patients with the same infection can be nursed together (cohorted) in one room, rather than in individual rooms (isolation).
Common law	The legal system developed over a period of time from old customs and court decisions, rather than laws made in Parliament.
Compensation	Monetary payment to compensate for loss or damage. It is also referred to as 'damages'.
Contemporaneously	Happening or existing at the same period of time.
Criminal law	The legal system that relates to punishing people who break the law.
Contraindication	A sign that someone should not continue with a particular medicine or treatment because it is, or might be, harmful.
CTG	Cardiotachograph is an electronic record in the form of a graph used to monitor the foetal heart rate during pregnancy.
Damages	Monetary payment to compensate for loss or damage. It is also referred to as compensation.

Defendant	A person in a law case who is accused of having done something unlawful.
Dermatologist	A doctor who studies and treats skin diseases.
Dermovate	A medication containing corticosteroid and used to decrease inflammation in the skin.
Duty of care	The legal obligation
Ectopic pregnancy	An ectopic pregnancy occurs when the fertilised egg attaches itself outside the cavity of the uterus (womb). The majority of ectopic pregnancies are found in the Fallopian tubes.
Employment tribunal	A legal process to hear and rule on disputes between employers and employees.
Fraud	A false representation by a statement or conduct in order to gain a material advantage.
Glomerulonephritis	The kidney's filters that continually reabsorb substances and remove waste from the blood become damaged and result in the kidney's inability to function
GMC	General Medical Council is the professional body for doctors.
House of Lords	The highest appeal court in England and Wales.
Inquest	A court process to discover the cause of someone's death.
Intrapartum	In the womb; referring to when the foetus is still in the womb.
Law Reports	Reports of cases decided by the courts.
Litigation	The process of taking a case to a law court so that an official decision can be made.
Man of straw	Someone with no money.
Myeloma	Cancer of white blood cells (called plasma cells). The cancerous plasma cells build up in the bone marrow.
Negligence	Failure to do something a reasonable person would do, or doing something that a reasonable person would not do. Where someone has a special skill, (e.g. a nurse), the person is expected to show the skill of the ordinary skilled nurse. Breach of the duty of care is also referred to as negligence.

NHSLA	National Health Service Legal Authority.
NICE	National Institute for Health and Clinical Excellence is an independent organisation responsible for providing national guidance on promoting good health and preventing and treating ill health.
NMC	Nursing and Midwifery Council is the professional body for nurses and midwives.
No win no fee	An agreement where legal costs will not be recovered by a solicitor if a claim for compensation is unsuccessful.
PDA	Personal Digital Assistant. Small, mobile handheld device that features computing, emailing and storage of information.
Pemphigoid	An autoimmune disease that causes blistering of the skin.
Postnatal	After the baby has been born.
Primary Care Trust	(PCTs) provide primary care services, which are the first point of call for a patient (e.g. GP practices, pharmacists, dentists and opticians). The PCTs also manage community services, such as district nursing, community hospitals and clinics.
Psoriasis	A chronic, recurring skin disease that causes one or more raised, red patches that have silvery scales and a distinct border between the patch and normal skin.
Recklessness	Doing something dangerous and not caring about the risks and the possible results.
Rigor	Sudden attack of severe shivering with feeling of coldness indicating a sudden worsening of a fever.
Standard of proof	Establishing the facts to the satisfaction of the court. The standard of proof in criminal proceedings is beyond reasonable doubt. The standard of proof in civil proceedings is on the balance of probabilities.
Statute	Act of parliament.

Sue	Take legal action against a person or organisation by making a legal claim for money because of some harm that they have caused.
TEN	Toxic epidermal necrolysis (TEN) is a life-threatening skin disease that cause rash, skin peeling, and sores on the mucous membranes.
Theft	Dishonestly taking property belonging to another.
Tort	A wrongful act or omission for which compensation can be claimed.
Trespass	A wrongful direct interference with another person or with their property.
Vicarious liability	Legal liability imposed on one person or organisation for the torts or crimes of another. Usually an employer is vicariously liable for its employees.

Index